Prevent

Cancer

Evidence-based Ways to Help Prevent Cancer Formation

(How a Heart-healthy Diet Can Prevent You against Cancer)

Gary Gonzalez

Published By **Oliver Leish**

Gary Gonzalez

All Rights Reserved

Prevent Cancer: Evidence-based Ways to Help Prevent Cancer Formation (How a Heart-healthy Diet Can Prevent You against Cancer)

ISBN   978-0-9959965-4-0

No part of this guidebook shall be reproduced in any form without permission in writing from the publisher except in the case of brief quotations embodied in critical articles or reviews.

Legal & Disclaimer

The information contained in this book is not designed to replace or take the place of any form of medicine or professional medical advice. The information in this book has been provided for educational & entertainment purposes only.

The information contained in this book has been compiled from sources deemed reliable, and it is accurate to the best of the Author's knowledge; however, the Author cannot guarantee its accuracy and validity and cannot be held liable for any errors or omissions. Changes are periodically made to this book. You must consult your doctor or get professional medical advice before using any of the suggested remedies, techniques, or information in this book.

Table Of Contents

Chapter 1: Your Body Is The Great Doctor With God's Power.

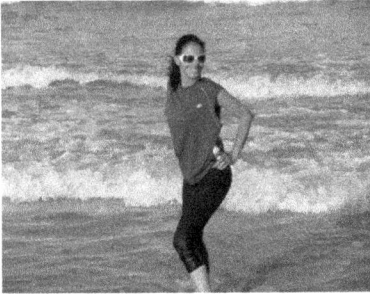

AS ALL LIFE COMES FROM GOD

The way that our bodies work is amazing. When you are sick your immune system starts to work in order to return their health. If you cut your arm, no

Doctors heal the cut and the body heals it. Our bodies are made by trillions of cells. And each one has an important purpose. White blood cells in our bodies are the soldiers of OUR body. They fight off viruses, bacteria and cancerous cells. and eliminate them in order in order to ensure that we are in good health. There are various kinds of blood-forming cells called white having different roles such as one kind of white blood cell known as neutrophil. It kills the fungus and bacteria, and can last from 6 hours up to days. To keep things as simple, for now, we'll use the same term for all varieties of white blood cells.

A variety of factors can weaken or reduce your immune system of the body including a poor nutrition, lack of exercise, stress, or insufficient water intake, etc. These and other factors can weaken our immune system, and make it not able to maintain our health.

"So the key to preventing cancer is to keep our body's immune system high so that our body can fight and destroy cancer cells". This is a short narrative to show the things I've written. Your friend and you are visiting someone who's suffering from an illness. There are a lot of microbes that are in the air, which both of you are breathing. Two days

Later, you learn later that the friend you took along with you for a visit is also suffering from a cold. You don't, for what reason? Your body's immune system is functioning perfectly there was plenty of white blood cells that could fight and eliminate cold-related bacteria that entered your body when you visited the acquaintance. The immune system of the friend was in decline, (insufficient white blood cells) as a result of the poor diet, stress levels and stress. The white blood cells couldn't cope with the task of eliminating bacteria that caused colds, and your client ended up getting an illness.

This book about Preventing Cancer you will be getting information on a myriad of things you can do to ensure that your immune system is well-maintained to avoid getting cancer, and to stay healthy.

Chapter 2: What Is Cancer ?

The cause of cancer is the consequence of cells that inexplicably expand and don't end up dying. The body's normal cells have a predictable path to development, division, and then death. Cell death that is programmed occurs as the apoptosis process, and once the process ceases and cancer develops, it can begin to grow. Contrary to normal cells that are normal cells, cancer cells don't undergo apoptosis, but instead remain growing and divisive. It results in a massive accumulation of cells with abnormalities that multiply beyond control. It can cause harm to the body as damaged cells grow in uncontrolled ways, forming lumps or massive masses of tissue referred to as tumors, except in cases of leukemia. In this case, cancer hinders normal blood flow through uncontrolled cell division within the bloodstream . In the event that a tumor spreads across the body and expands, taking over and damaging the healthy tissue around it It is believed to be metastasized. The term used to describe this process is metastasis.

What results is a severe disease that's very difficult to manage. The most common cause of death for cancer patients is metastasis. Tumors are

usually treatable, provided they do not have moved into vital organs.

There are more than 100 cancer types that impact diverse parts of our bodies. Every type of cancer has distinct causes, signs as well as treatment options. Similar to all types of illness, there are certain kinds of cancer have a higher prevalence in comparison to others.

Common Types of Cancer

Breast cancer, bladder cancer and colon cancer. Endometrial cancer kidney cancer) Leukemia, lung cancer, melanoma and non-Hodgkin lymphoma and pancreatic cancer thyroid cancer of the prostate as well as skin cancer.

The year 1901 was the first time cancer was recognized as an uncommon disease. Research shows that only 1 of 8000 people had been diagnosed with cancer. According to the American Cancer Society, 1 out of three will be diagnosed with cancer.

1 338 910 people have been confirmed to have the disease.

cancers was a major cause of death in cancer in the U.S. in 2012. The cancers that were diagnosed claimed the lives of 577,190 which is about one-third of the patients diagnosed with cancer.

More than 1500 deaths occur each more than 1,500 deaths per. Lung cancers and bronchus as well as prostate as well as colorectal, in men, as well as cancers of the lung and bronchus as well as breast and colorectal among women are still the top causes of cancer deaths. These four types of cancer represent nearly 50% of the deaths from cancer in both genders.

SIGNS OF POSSIBLE CANCER YOU NEED TO BE AWARE OF.

An area of lumpy tissue in your body.

Moles that change shape in the skin (such as itching, bleeding or changes in color or shape).

Hoarseness or a cough that persists for longer than 2 weeks.

An alteration in the way you eat lasting for longer than 2 weeks.

Atypical bleeding that occurs from the vagina, colon or even within your urine, or during you are vomiting.

Astonishingly weight loss that is not explained (10 pounds. in a few months).

Chapter 3: Genetics Of Cancer

Genetics is a factor in our lives since the moment we are born. It decides what we sex as well as our height, the colour of our eyes and our intelligence level and so on. It also affects the likelihood of developing many ailments, like cancer.

Genetic information is a way to determine if someone is at a higher risk of getting cancer. Genetic information sources comprise DNA from biological samples and information from the family history of a person's of cancer, the results of physical examinations and medical documents.

Cancer is a very common illness that it's very common for families to contain at the very least family members with cancer. Sometime, specific types of cancer are seen to be prevalent within certain families. It could be due to many reasons. In most cases, families share specific risk factors like smoking which may cause a range of types of cancer. However, in certain instances cancers are caused by an unnatural gene transferred from one generation to generations. Though this can be called inherited cancer, the fact that it is passed down is

The abnormal gene may cause cancer but not actually the cancer. The majority of 10% of cancers are caused by inheritance.

If someone is born with an abnormal copy of the gene, the cells have just one mutation. This makes it simpler (and faster) for a sufficient number of mutations to form so that a cell can develop into cancer. This is the reason why cancers that have a genetic basis tend to manifest sooner than cancers similar to them which aren't inherited.

What should I be concerned about?

Certain circumstances increase the likelihood that an abnormal gene could be responsible for causing family-wide cancers like

There are many instances of a rare or uncommon form of cancer (like kidney cancer).

* Some cancers are diagnosed at earlier years than the norm (like colon cancer that occurs in 20-year old)

* There are more than one kind of cancer can occur in one individual (like women who have two types of cancer - ovarian and breast).

* The cancers can be found within the organs (both eyes the kidneys and both eyes, as well as each breast).

* There is more than one childhood cancer within a group of siblings (like Sarcomas in the case of a brother as well as a sister).

If you are deciding that the family has a history of cancer Begin by gathering details. In each instance of cancer, consider:

Who's in the affected group? What are the ramifications?

* What kind of cancer? Are they uncommon?

* What was the age of this particular relative when it was diagnosed?

Did this person have several types of cancer?

* Do they smoke cigarettes or had other risks?

A close relative with cancer similar to sibling or parent (brother or sibling) can be a cause to be concerned than cancer that occurs that occurs in distant relatives. If the cancer resulted caused by a genetic mutation and it is possible for it to pass on, the likelihood of being passed on to your children is smaller with the more distant family members.

The results of studies have revealed that those with genetic traits when they live an ideal life style, they are less likely to get cancer.

Chapter 4: A Healthy Diet

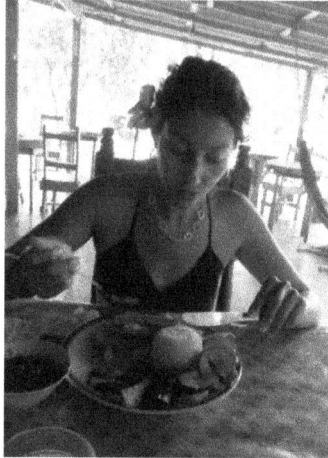

The information you find in this chapter could make you think twice about the foods is the best food to eat in order in order to remain healthy and avoid cancer. We are all aware that we have to eat more healthy organic foods, and fewer refined ones in order to remain clear of cancer. We are taking a look at what foods we need to eat and the foods we shouldn't be eating.

WHAT WE SHOULD BE EATING TO PREVENT CANCER

There is no one diet or food that will protect you against cancer. However, making a small change to the way you eat can cut down the likelihood of getting cancer by a third. Certain foods actually can fight cancer by blocking the creation of carcinogens responsible for cancer, as well as preventing the carcinogens from reaching vital organs. Some foods prevent cells exposed to cancer-causing substances from developing cancerous. Others help to heal cancerous regions of the body.

The first step to making your own personal fight against cancer is choosing the diet which is high in fiber, and lower in fat. It should also is packed with fresh fruits as well as vegetables. According to the National Cancer Institute suggests that Americans consume five or more portions of fruit and vegetables each day. They also recommend 6 to 11 portions of

grains as depicted in grain, as depicted on U.S. Department of Agriculture food pyramid. The daily consumption between 20 and 30 grams of fiber in fruit, vegetables cereals, whole grains as well as dried beans and peas is suggested.

Here's a summary of the most important cancer-fighting foods that you should include in your daily diet on a consistent routine

Garlic is one of the most popular foods. Garlic has a variety of substances that be protective against cancer, specifically ones of the skin the colon and lung.

Turmeric prevents and reduces the development of several forms of cancer, notably cancers of the esophagus stomach, mouth, intestines the breast and even the skin.

Dark Leafy Greens - Dark Greens are an excellent source of antioxidants, also known as carotenoids. They remove harmful free radicals in the body, before they are able to increase the growth of cancer.

Grapes - Grapes have the chemical resveratrol. This is an extremely potent antioxidant which could stop the cell from being damaged before it starts.

Tomatoes contain the chemical compound lycopene (which is the most readily absorbable from tomatoes cooked) has been proven to reduce the risk of prostate cancer along with cancers of the lung, breast and stomach.

Blueberries: Of all fruit, blueberries rank as the most potent in fighting cancer chemicals. They can aid in the treatment of every type of cancer.

Cruciferous vegetables - Vegetables such as cauliflower, broccoli, cabbage, as well as Brussels sprouts have antioxidants, which may reduce the risk of developing cancer.

Whole Grains: Whole grains are a source of various compounds that fight cancer such as antioxidants, fiber as well as phytoestrogens.

They can reduce the likelihood of developing all kinds of cancer.

All Types of Raw Fruits and Vegetables -

It is recommended eating more fresh fruit and vegetables since they have more minerals, vitamins and chemicals than foods cooked. Raw vegetables and fruits also contain enzymes, which have lost in cooking. The most significant ingredient they have is what called the life force, something that science hasn't yet discovered. If you pick a seed and boil it, before planting it, it will never expand, but if you use the similar seed uncooked and put it in the ground and the seed will begin to grow. This is because the seed contains the vital energy in it. Incorporate cancer cells in cooked food medium and they'll begin to expand. Then, place the cancerous cells in raw food medium and they'll disappear! Raw food that can kill cancer cells. That is the thing I refer to as the Life Force. It's a miracle!

This fact is well-known by that fact is known to the American Cancer Society, but it was not reported to the general public. Therefore, it's crucial to eat plenty of fresh fruits and vegetables.

I usually avoid writing about negative stuff, however this article that you're about see is a different story. Because I mentioned my experience with the American Cancer Society I feel it is my duty to tell my readers some information regarding this organization. American Cancer Society. The organization doesn't want the cure of cancer. Instead, they do their best to denigrate those seeking an answer. In the past, they had declared that eating a healthy diet did not have anything to do with contribute to the development of cancer. In the end, they had to alter their beliefs, and why? Because different organizations like The National Cancer Institute did the research to show the fact that eating habits can cause cancer. Now, they are American Cancer Society says we should eat more fruit and vegetables in order to reduce the risk of cancer. The society was forced to alter their mind. I'm sorry they did not use part of the money they get to discover the cure for cancer based on research that shows that a bad nutrition can lead to cancer. The other group needed to perform the same task as they did. American Cancer Society was founded to accomplish. There are many other organizations, including that of the American Medical Association that is working in the same way similar to what it is the American Cancer Society does. We are not looking for the cure to cancer. This is an investigation conducted in the Journal of the American Medical Association which

It's not even research. The study was conducted in 2005 and they concluded that the diet doesn't have any influence on cancer.

Do Fruits and Vegetables Prevent Cancer?

A study published at the beginning of 2005 by The Journal of the American Medical Association discovered that there is no link between eating fruit and vegetables with the likelihood of developing breast cancer. Do you believe this? What is the relationship between this and the "big picture" of what we have learned about cancer and diet?

What was the subject of research?

The researchers first found no differences in the rate of breast cancer, in women who ate just 114 grams of daily fruit with those who had reported eating 367 g or more of fruits every day.

To give you an idea, a moderate apple weighs approximately 250 grams. Also the comparison of people who consume more than 114 grams of fruit every day to those who consume 367 grams of fruit each day would be like comparing individuals eating half of a medium-sized apple per day to people taking one big daily apple. This study did not show any benefit to having fruit when researchers examined women who consume around one half to one portion of fruit daily against women

• eating between two and three portions of fruit a every day.

There is the same as studies have demonstrated that we require at least five portions of vegetables and fruits daily to fight cancer. This is not only one apple. It's amazing that they could claim this is a study of science.

WHAT WE SHOULD NOT BE EATING TO PREVENT CANCER.

It's impossible to list all harmful substances found in refined foods, therefore in this article I will discuss the detrimental impacts of eggs, meat as well as dairy products, sugar and meat because I believe they are the ingredients that are most dangerous in creating cancer. In the past, you've read 3 out of every 4 Americans suffer from cancer. one reason for this is that the American diet is primarily comprised of eggs, meat as well as dairy products, sugar and. In 2002, the median intake of meat per person was 250 lbs. Most recent statistics show that the overall milk consumption which covers all varieties of dairy is 506 pounds. per person in a year. In 2009, egg consumption per person was around 250 eggs annually. The most common sugar consumption per individual for the year was 107 lbs. Today we are able to understand one of the causes that one in three Americans dies from cancer.

DIET IS THE MAJOR CAUSE OF DISEASE

A report of 712 pages, released from the U.S. The Surgeon General, in 1979 (today we don't have the U.S. Surgeon General presenting these kinds of information because he's subordinate to those in high-ranking posts). This report from 1979 cites over 2,000 studies across the globe and, on the advice of over 200 doctors or nutritionists as well as biochemists. They reached the conclusion that the typical American diet could be dangerous. Out of those 2.1 million Americans that died, in the study, 1.5 million were killed by ailments that were caused by eating habits. It was revealed the need to reduce intake of fats and saturated fats for example, eggs the butter, or red meat that is not cut. It recommends greater consumption of fruits and vegetables and more whole grain food items and cereal products. It recommends dried legumes, like peas, and beans are utilized as sources of protein, to supplement animals' food items. The report said that consuming fats from the diet noted, can increase the risk of being overweight and certain types of cancer the gallbladder, heart disease, and other cancers. In addition, the report recommended that excessive cholesterol levels, which are strongly linked in heart attacks need to be diminished by restricting consumption of products with animals, like eggs milk products, dairy, chicken, meat and fish.

The report of the surgeon general suggests that we cut down on the consumption of animal products as well as other animal-based foods including eggs, as well as dairy-based products. I'm sure that the dairy and meat industries weren't happy with the report. If I were to take this one step further and believe it is best to eliminate these products out of our diet as fast as we can.

Cancer Facts - Meat Consumption and Cancer Risk

It is believed that the World Health Organization has determined that diet-related factors are responsible for a minimum of 33 percent of cancers found in Western countries, and as high as 20 percent in countries that are developing. As cancer researchers began to look for a link between food and cancer among the most notable results was that those who ate less meat were more likely to avoid developing cancer. Numerous studies conducted from England as well as Germany found that vegetarians were approximately 40 percent less likely get cancer when compared with people who consume meat.

Harvard researchers conducted an analysis prospectively of 90,655 women who were premenopausal, between the ages of 26 and 46 who were enrolled as part of the Nurses' Health Study II and found that consumption of animal fats, specifically from red meats and high-fat dairy products, in women who are premenopausal is associated with the risk of developing breast cancer.

Similar to breast cancer the consumption of meat frequently especially red meat can increase the chance of developing colon cancer.

Prostate Cancer

Prostate cancer is among the most prevalent cancers in males across the U.S., and researchers have investigated a range of possible factors in the diet that contribute to

prostate cancer risk. This includes dietary fats saturated fat dairy products, meat. They also include food items that can reduce risk of developing prostate cancer, like eating carotenoids, various antioxidants. They also include fiber as well as fruit. In the same way as breast cancer risks men's consumption of fats in the diet that is found in abundance in meats and other animal products (dairy as well as eggs) can increase testosterone levels, which is in turn, increases the risk of prostate cancer.

A Yale study showed that women who consumed highest amount of animal protein were at an increased risk of 70 percent of developing non-Hodgkin's lymphoma which is a cancer of the lymphoid tissues, which include those lymph nodes spleen as well as various other parts of the immune system.

What we've just seen in the previous paragraphs is clearly evident and study of science confirms that vegetarians have the lowest chance for developing cancer. They also have an extremely low risk of developing cancer in comparison to those who eat meat.

THE ANIMAL KINGDOM IS DISEASED AND DANGEROUS TO CONSUME

It's just one of the examples I'd like to give you. You may recall that on the 11th of March, 2011 the strongest earthquake that ever struck Japan created a tsunami, with waves up to up to 144 feet. These

The waves flooded waves flooded the Fukushima nuclear power-plant complex creating a complete shutdown that led to the most devastating nuclear event since the 1986 Chernobyl catastrophe. The incident has been classified as an '7' on a scale from 1-7 according to the International Nuclear Event Scale. The cooling water that is contaminated has been released directly into the sea and has made its way into the ecosystem. The water from storage tanks is also leaking into groundwater before flowing to the ocean. The efforts to put in place a variety of barriers to avoid pollution haven't completely stopped the loss.

"The quantities of water they are dealing with are absolutely gigantic," stated Mycle Schneider, a non-profit consultant who previously worked with the French as well as the German governments, and consulted frequently for many organisations and nations concerning nuclear concerns. "What is worse is the water leakage everywhere else - not just from the tanks. It is leaking out from the basements, it is leaking out from the cracks all over the place. Nobody can measure that."

As per Maxim Shingarkin, deputy chairman of Russia's State Duma Committee for Natural Resources, "Currents in the world ocean are so structured that the areas of seafood capture near the U.S. northwest coast are more likely to contain radioactive nuclides than even the Sea of Okhotsk, which is much closer to Japan. These products are the main danger for mankind because they can find their way to people's tables on a massive scale."

The issue is important for this country United States since, according to the National Marine Fisheries Service, the U.S. imported almost 45 million pounds of fish from Japan in 2012. It's clear that the consequences of this catastrophe remain a long way off.

Man's Body Was Not Designed To Eat Meat.

Let's take a look at the basic physical aspects of eating meat. Carnivores' teeth are extremely sharp, long with a pointed tip for cutting and breaking flesh. Humans have molars that are used that crush and grind. Carnivores' jaws move upwards and downwards only to bite and tear. Man's tongue moves upwards and downwards and side-to-side to grind. Carnivores' tongues are rough, while man's tongue is.

smooth. The saliva of carnivores is acidic and specifically designed for digestion of protein from animals. The saliva of man is alkaline to the digestion of protein.

digestive process of the starch. Carnivores' intestines measure three times longer than its trunk. It is designed for the rapid elimination of food items that would otherwise decay. The intestines of a man are 12 times longer than the trunk, and are designed to maintain

Chapter 5: Fresh Air And Pure Water

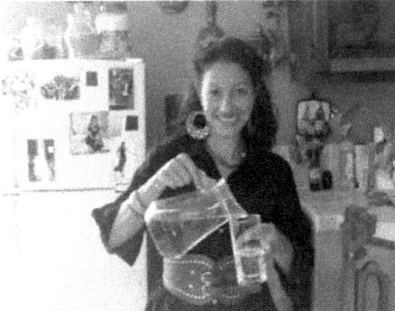

FRESH AIR AND PURE WATER

The most basic need for all living things on planet is oxygen. The living creatures cannot exist without oxygen. Oxygen is always found in every breath that we breathe. The trillions of cells that make up the human body

The body needs to receive a continuous flow of oxygen, or cells will begin to shrink and die.

AIR IS ELECTRICALLY CHARGED

Air contains electricity. The air we breathe influences the body in the same way as if it was charged with electric current. This electric energy, which is absorption by blood, is transmitted to every part in the body. Air we breathe is a source of negative charged ions, as well as positively charged ones. Our bodies require a bigger amount of negatively charged ions to ensure optimal well-being. Inhaling large quantities of positively charged particles (the bad ones) and experience these negative side effects, such like nasal obstruction, headache as well as hoarseness, fatigue dizziness, dry throat and so on. The air that is mostly negative charged (the positive kind) produces feeling of happiness and exhilaration. Air that is negatively charged (the best type) can be found near the ocean or in mountains near the base of a waterfall, or along streams or rivers. The air we breathe outside has lots of positive negative ions. That's why it is so enjoyable whenever we camp or go to the sea. If one feels tired, taking a walk out in the fresh air is sure to rejuvenate your whole body. It is estimated that there are three to 4000 positive negative ions within one cubic centimeter of mountain air yet only one hundred negative ions within one cubic centimeter of air inside an office space towards the end of an 8-hour workday. In enclosed buildings, there are a lot of negative positively charged ions that are dangerous to the health. Every electrical appliance such as air conditioners, and so on. utilize the beneficial negative ions, and release negative ions that are harmful. The air we breathe is negatively charged which is why one is drowsy after spending many hours in a room which is crowded with individuals. You wouldn't think of having a meal that someone else has chewed. Yet, people don't know that breath in a confined, toxic air for a long time can cause blood poisoning and harm the lungs. For good health, our houses should provide adequate ventilation (windows are open during the winter as well as summer). Modern, airtight home and air conditioning systems which circulate large amounts of our indoor pollutants and allowing us to breathe,

Our lungs are not getting enough clean, fresh air. The oxygen that our bodies get through the air is crucial in maintaining healthy and in good well-being. In the absence of air and fresh air, vital task of adjusting blood's chemistry would not be accomplished successfully and the person would be suffering severe effects.

OXYGEN KILLS CANCER CELLS

Cancer cells are not able to exist in a state of oxygen that is positively charged and good. If they are exposed to oxygen, they cease to live. It is a sign that we must take a deep breath of the fresh air of our country. It is known that oxygen comprises 21% of earth's atmospheric air, however researchers have observed that oxygen concentrations have decreased to below 15% in the metropolitan areas.

Doctor. Otto Warburg, was a biochemist working on the field of cancer research. He received the Nobel Prize in Medicine for showing that cancer cells can't exist within an unoxidized, healthy cell. The doctor. Warburgh was the director of the Max Planck Institute for Cell Physiology in Germany. In

"The Prime Cause and Prevention of Cancer" 1967,

The Dr. Warburg proposed that normalizing the metabolic process of cancer cells was essential for a successful treatment of cancer. The way for achieving this was by increasing the amount of oxygen in the cells. The Dr. Warburg stated that as the primary goal of the treatment "-- all growing body cells be saturated with oxygen" and that the next prioritization was to prevent any further exposure to toxic substances.

NATURAL WAYS TO PURIFY AIR

A natural method to clean the air inside your office or home is to keep plenty of plants that live, as they absorb carbon dioxide we inhale and transform it into oxygen. A single plant can remove as much as 87% of the toxins within 100 square feet each day. Therefore, if your house or office area is 2500 square. feet. in area, you'd have to plant 20 trees throughout your office or house.

Following my article on the role of the freshness of air in fighting cancer, I am hoping my readers are inspired to begin spending longer outdoors in clean air, and using their air conditioners as much as is possible, and also making sure that they have a partially-open window in their bedroom.

PURE WATER

WHAT IS PURE SOFT WATER?

Apart from pure air, there's any other natural element which is as vital for sustaining life like purified soft water. The chemical makeup of pure soft water can be characterized in the formula chemical H20. This means that it's made up of two hydrogen parts and one element oxygen. It is colorless, odorless tasting, transparent and tasteless without any minerals or chemical inside it.

Where can we find pure soft water in this era of chemical pollution? The municipal water supply has been discovered to have more than 700 chemical compounds, but federal laws mandate tests for just 16 of them. New research suggests that the chemical chlorine, utilized by municipal water sources to kill bacteria is more hazardous for health in humans than initially believed to be. It's been proven to play a major role for certain cancers and heart diseases. It is important to note that if you are required to drink water with chlorinated elements, have it put out in a clean container or in the fridge for a short duration before drinking it since the chlorine in the water and vaporizes in the air.

Unforgettable warnings about tap water. Many people believe that their municipality is accountable for providing them with drinking water that is safe to drink. It's not the case. The federal courts have ruled that cities can not be held accountable for the quality and purity of the water it consumes. . There are at least 6,000 cases of bladder cancer, and around more than 8,000 instances of

rectal cancers that occur in Rectal Cancer that is reported in United States each year may occur as a direct consequence of drinking water that is chlorinated. It is imperative to go at a different source of water as just half of

less than one percent of household water is used to drink as well as for cooking.

Do you have bottled water?

WASHINGTON (October 15th (October 15) - - Ten well-known U.S. bottles of water include a mix of 38 distinct pollutants, including bacteria fertilizers, Tylenol and industrial chemicals with some levels barely higher than tap water in the latest laboratory tests carried out by the Environmental Working Group (EWG).

Walmart's Sam's Choice at several locations had contaminants higher than California's bottle standards for water quality as well as safe levels of carcinogens as per the California's Safe Drinking Water and Toxic Enforcement Act. Giant Food's Acadia brand has consistently maintained the highest concentrations of cancer-causing chlorine byproducts in the suburbs of Washington DC tap water from the source of its production.

And where can we buy Pure soft water?

MINERALS IN WATER ARE HARMFUL TO YOUR HEALTH !

Inorganic water is composed of minerals that are not absorbed in the human body. The only minerals that the body can absorb can be absorbed by the body are organic minerals. Inorganic minerals need to be removed or else they could eventually cause health issues. There's a significant contrast between the iron that is powdered, (inorganic iron), as well as the iron that is found in plant matter like spinach (organic iron). If we drink hard water that is enriched with magnesium, calcium or iron, copper silicon and so on. We do not think about the fact that our bodies are incapable of absorbing

These inorganic minerals. The mineral deposits can be found in joints due to arthritis, within the intestinal wall causing constipation, as well as in the arteries, causing the formation of

harden. The kidneys enlarge mineral deposits and form small stones called kidney stones. They grow until they are to large enough to fit into the valves. Heart valves and chambers may be so firmly bonded with mineral deposits that surgery for the heart may be required.

DISTILLED WATER AND REVERSE OSMOSIS WATER ARE PURE SOFT WATERS

Distilled water refers to water that is heated before being transformed into vapor so it is almost entirely contaminants are eliminated because they're incapable of converting into a liquid. After that, the vapors of water get cooled and you are left with distilled water. Distilled water is tasteless and free of or color. It also does not smell and is free of heavy metals, bacteria acid and inorganic minerals, harmful chemicals, poisons and so on. Rainwater is also distilled, however it is polluted when it flies through the air and is therefore pure water. One simple way to test this at home is boiling an unopened pan of tap water. Allow it to boil until the water is turned into little vapor. What remains in the pan's bottom pot? If the water is packed with minerals, you'll be able to see white chalky mineral deposits at the pan's bottom. The harder water is, contains minerals, the higher amount it will comprise; and the less minerals, the more soft the water. Distilled water does not contain any minerals, therefore it's only soft and pure water. Another filter that is equivalent to distillers that provides soft, pure water, and costs less to run than a distiller is an Reverse Osmosis filtering unit that can also eliminate all the contaminants in the water.

Chapter 6: Sunshine Fights Cancer

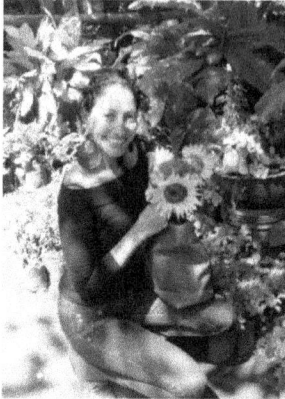

For the majority of recorded time the human race has lived and worked outside, with total exposure to the sun. Today, in our society many people live in city, working inside offices and factories. Our lives are in glass-based environments, and much of our time is covered by glass windows and blocks away the UV light that can be so beneficial to the body. Light sources such as incandescent or fluorescent are employed in workplaces, schools and in factories. The light source used is completely distinct from the light that is derived from daylight. Natural sunlight in its full, direct form is as intense at 10,000 foot candles. However, the highest intensity of an fluorescent fixture with the equivalent of ten tubes with an 8 foot diameter can be as low as 1,000 foot candles spread over the distance of 10-12 inches.

SUNSHINE FIGHTS CANCER !

The sun's rays can accelerate the metabolism of your body in order to flush out toxic toxins your body accumulates. The UV light assists in get rid of these. In turn, by helping in the elimination of many cancer-causing agents, the sun helps to decrease the risk of developing cancer. Research has shown that when the quantity of sunlight available is increased, the likelihood of cancers in the internal organs is reduced. Sunshine increases the usage of oxygen within tissues. This is crucial for stimulating the immune system specifically in the generation of antibodies. There are many kinds of

The cancerous cells don't enjoy oxygen, so when they are exposed to high levels of oxygen, cancer cells will slow the growth of their cells and divide and eventually stop completely within

In this manner, indirect sunlight could combat cancer by increasing the immune system's effectiveness as well as increasing the amount of oxygen that is absorbed by tissues.

CAN SUNLIGHT CAUSE CANCER?

Certain people are extremely sensitive to light and can be easily burned. People with red and blonde hair are the most likely to suffer by chronic burning. Skin cancer sufferers seem to be extremely susceptible to the sun's rays. The sun burns them more frequently and their burns can take longer to recover. Also, they have a tougher time getting tan. According to the current medical theory, there is the sun as a destructive one, which is responsible for ageing of the skin as well as producing skin cancer. The research that is based on this idea gives information about the sun's role and relationship to health of humans. Undoubtedly, the sun plays an important role in the development of the development of skin cancers and ageing however is it actually the main cause? The Dr. Zane Kime M.D. who is the author of Sunlight Could Save Your Life gained more conviction when he analyzed the available studies, which showed that a refined Western diet, particularly one made is based on refined oils plays major roles in the growth of skin cancer. He also discovered the sun's rays only cause the issue to worsen. Salad and cooking oil has risen drastically since 1909 when cooking oils were consumed at a rate of 1.5 pounds per person each year. In the present, that number exceeds 70 pounds for each person. There's no doubt according to research, about whether the consumption of high-fat foods leads to an earlier and higher rate of skin problems.

The cause of cancer is the ultraviolet radiation. Skin cancer is not the only one as well, but colon and breast cancers as well, are thought to be accelerated by the consumption of a fat-rich diet through indirect means.

sunshine can combat cancer by activating the immune system and boosting the amount of oxygen that is in the tissues. Vitamin D and sun exposure are connected. The sun's rays on skin produce certain hormones as well as nutrients such as Vitamin D. If one does not is eating a healthy diet, sunlight can have a negative effect upon the face. The following must be noted: sunlight bathing can be dangerous especially for people who follow the Standard fat-rich American diet (which contains 45percent fat) or don't have a sufficient intake of fruits, vegetables, whole grains as well as fresh fruit. This isn't just the diet-related fats that cause the development of skin cancer and spread, but also the fat from oil that is applied directly on the skin. That's why sun-bath creams, lotions, or even oils aren't advised, as they could cause cancer to develop. Also, sunscreens that I discuss in my chapter on chemical exposure.

Chapter 7: Getting Sufficient Rest

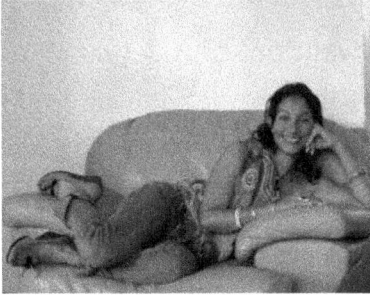

The concept of rest is among the most fundamental healers that have been discovered by mankind. When you get unwell, what's the first step you take? In bed all day long in addition to throughout the night until you heal, since the power of rest is vital to wellness. Each bodily muscle needs rest following exertion. The heart, the most powerful muscle working that you have every time you beat. It rests at the end of every breath. Your muscles require relaxation after every contraction. In the evening, the body's repair process is on. The most enthusiastic people I have met are very regular in their sleep. One reason to rest is to heal damages and injuries resulted from work.

Since the invention of television, a lot of people aren't getting enough sleep. They fall asleep late and wake up early for work, and then in the middle of the day, they must force themselves to go on.

Make time to review your day; allow yourself to take a break. Sit outside in a recliner and do nothing. If that is a bit scary to you, that's the person who should change your mindset towards a restful sleep.

HOW MUCH SLEEP DO WE NEED?

The need for rest varies as you get older. The baby is asleep most of all the time. Children who are young prior to age 6 requires about 14 hours of sleeping every day. The average grade school student must sleep at least 12 hours, and teenagers should have a sleep time of nine or the tenth hour of every daily. It is not required for adults However, it's essential ideal for children. Adults are not required to sleep.

requires only the repair of everyday waste of tissues, the youthful require more energy to support the growth and development. Yet, studies show that people who are good at sleeping among older people are the ones who last the longest. It is possible that sleep requirements change. With pregnancy, illness, or stressful times, someone might require more rest. In the event that worries, fears and business worries get put to bed and sleep is not a pleasant experience, the morning hours isn't rejuvenating and the amount of rest is usually prolonged. Working in the day also affects how much sleep you get during the evening. People who work with the brain, as well as those who are suffering from severe nerve strains require a significant amount of rest: their stress is neurological and mental and sleeping is the sole form of relaxation that can be advantageous. Workers who do manual tasks, tend to go easily to sleep upon retirement and do not require more than a few hours of rest.

NATURAL WAYS TO HELP ONE SLEEP

.

The only people who work their muscles throughout the day working out can experience the sweet rest of their nights. If you're a sitting person, after dinner, you should spend at minimum one hour outdoors, take walks, mow your lawn, wash your car, take a walk in the garden, or paint your garage or garage, etc. Or do some work prior to going to go to bed.

It is essential to maintain regular sleeping routines. Aiming to wake up in the same way each day will aid to fall asleep at the exact time each at night. Making bed in the early hours is extremely beneficial to one's wellbeing. There is evidence that body temperature and vitality are at their lowest point around 2

A.M. This is the reason, every hour of rest before midnight is worth 2 hours. Likewise, every minute after midnight counts for one hour.

Tobacco or caffeine (as present in tea, coffee and the colas) sugar, chocolate fats, chemicals used in additives, preservatives and additives. could stimulate the body, causing sleepiness.

Food can make you sleepy in the beginning, because it draws the head's blood however, it can disturb sleeping later on in the night. If you consume a huge breakfast prior to sleeping in the evening, your food needs to be digested, and the stomach is unable to receive the proper amount of relaxation. It is a disturbance to sleep as the nerves and brain fatigued, appetite to eat breakfast suffers and your entire body isn't well-rested and in no condition to perform the tasks of the day.

Chapter 8: Exercise For Cancer Prevention

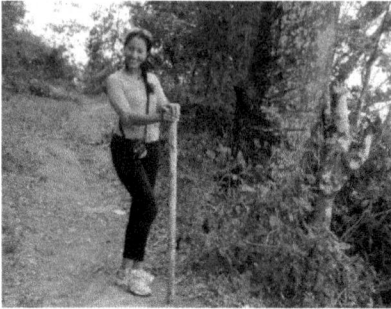

Do you realize that if you exercise, you're less likely to be a victim of different forms of cancer?

It is recommended that the American Cancer Society recommends exercising for 30 minutes minimum 5 times a week, to help prevent cancer. It doesn't mean attending the gym in order to work out. There are many ways to incorporate exercise into your routine. Regular exercise can keep us fit and, yes, helps fight many forms of cancers, like colon cancer. The large intestine of your body is sort of like a sewerage plant. It is able to recycle the substances that your body needs and then stores garbage for later elimination. As long as waste remains within the rectum or colon and the more toxic substances need to be eliminated from the stool that is solidifying and then back to the tissues. The exercise routine gets your body moving as well as getting the waste that is in your body moving. The reason for this is that exercise triggers peristalsis, which is a type of muscular contraction that assists in pushing the colon to eliminate waste. Studies have shown that exercise can reduce the risk of colon cancer by as much as 40 percent. Training also helps reduce the risk of risk factors that can cause colon cancer.

One of the most important positive effects of exercise on your health is that it aids in normalizing your insulin, glucose and leptin levels through optimizing the leptin receptor's sensitivity and insulin. It is arguably the primary aspect

to improve the overall health of your body and helping to avoid diseases that are chronic, which could help explain why exercise is an effective preventive medication. Recent research has have concluded that exercising can be "the best preventive drug" for a myriad of ailments such as psychiatric diseases, heart conditions as well as diabetes and cancer. The ideal place for the exercises is outside with the sunshine and fresh air. Exercise in a gym can be similar to exercising in a filthy tennis shoe.

Seven Exercises I would recommend for getting fit!

1. Walking is easy, all you require is a decent pair of footwear.

2. The only thing you require is a bathing suit.

3. Bicycling, and only you'll need an bicycle.

4. The push-ups can tone many muscles throughout the body and also get your heart rate up.

5. Set-Ups can be beneficial for back, stomach and back, as well as keeping your body looking slim and toned.

6. Squats can be beneficial for legs.

7. The ideal overall exercise that I would highly suggest, is to jump on the trampoline in miniature.

The exercise on this one is sure to work the most muscles of your body than other exercises. A mini trampoline is a great way to exercise all day long.

trillions of cells that make up your body move between a horizontal and a vertical plane, as are every cell inside your body. I

It is impossible to even begin to list all the organs and systems it assists however, we can mention just some of them, including the lungs, heart muscle, leg muscles and stomach muscles, back muscles and your balance. etc. The tramp is not harmful to joints of the body since it's not an activity that is a high impact like jogging. I would not suggest. For people who are old or have issues in balance, you can put an extra high-back chair in the middle of the mini tramp, and then hold the chair when you are jumping.

This is the best exercise to strengthen the lymphatic system. The body has approximately. 5 quarts blood inside our bodies. However, there are more than 10 tons of lymphatic fluid. The lymphatic system helps the immune system by destroying pathogens by removing excessive waste, fluid, debris and dead blood cells cancerous cells, pathogens and other harmful substances from these cells as well as the spaces between the cells. Additionally, it works alongside the circulatory system in order to supply oxygen, nutrients and hormones from blood to the tissues which make up the body's tissues. To stay fit, get started with the exercise !!!!! !

Naturally, we should be aware that excessive amounts of anything good can cause harm to our bodies including exercise.

Chapter 9: Dealing With Stress

75 percent of the population is experiencing at the very least "some stress" every two weeks (National Health

Interview Survey). The majority of respondents suffer from moderate or high levels of stress over the exact two-week time frame.

Many millions of Americans are suffering from excessive stress levels in their work environments. Stress is a major cause of cardiovascular disease, high blood pressure, strokes and a host of other diseases in many people. Stress affects also the immune system.

Our system shields us from a range of dangerous

conditions like cancer.

Stress can also lead to growth of obesity, alcoholism as well as suicide, addiction to drugs and smoking cigarettes.

addiction and other dangerous addiction, and other harmful. Stress is so common that it is the reason that U.S. Public Health Service has set a goal to reduce stress as among its top goals for health promotion.

SO HOW DO WE DEAL WITH STRESS?

The first step is to recognize the cause of stress. Second, you need to find solutions. Two instances: It is not your favorite job. So if are concerned about your mental peace

If you are concerned about your health, then it is time look at a new one , this may take some time however at the very least, you're headed towards the proper direction. The stress that you experience can control. However, this type of stress that you are unable to modify. For instance, if your partner suddenly passes away, that is the moment the issue to the higher power through prayers, mediation, etc.

In times of stress The adrenal glands inject adrenalin into bloodstream to provide the strength to fighting or fleeing. The adrenalin can be harmful for the body if it's not utilized. There are two things that I suggest doing during times of pressure. In the first place, drink plenty of water to aid in diluting the amount of adrenalin that exists in blood streams. Next, get outside and engage in any kind of activity to burn off the adrenalin that is in excess (read the chapter about the most effective kinds of exercises).

Are there any medications you can take to ease the anxiety? The medication will not solve the issue leading to the stress, which often times, makes it even much worse. There are many adverse negative effects, which usually slow everything that the body does like not being able to drive an automobile after having taken the medicine. These medications can cause other side effects too.

decrease your metabolism and you're overweight, suffer from little energy, can't think clearly, etc. Also, they weaken the immune system, which means you could develop an illness like cancer, or another.

Over many years, I've observed that a lot of my patients who were diagnosed with cancer typically were victims of a tragedy during their lives that caused stress before they were diagnosed with cancer.

If you're feeling stressed frustrated, sad, or unhappy. Drink a glass of water, then go outdoors and take an extended walk, then write your list, or consider everything you're grateful for. You are alive, are able to eat food and clothes to put on as well as loved ones who cherish your. etc. Following these steps, I'm sure that you'll feel more relaxed. Do it again and observe.

Chapter 10: Maintain A Positive And Happy Attitude

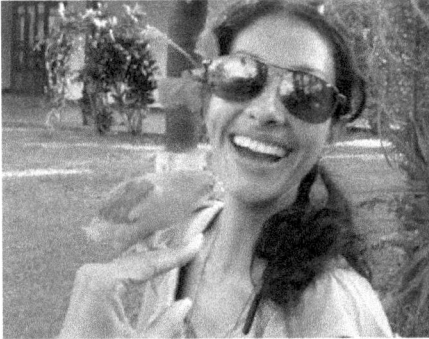

University of California researchers found actors can alter their immune systems due to the emotion they display. The research has been based on research done by universities like from Harvard, Duke University, University of Chicago, etc. that show a direct link with improved health, a longer lifespan, and happiness when one has an optimistic, positive attitude toward the world. The science behind mind-body medicine has been confirmed scientifically," says Herbert Benson who is a cardiologist and medical professor within Harvard Medical School who is known as a pioneer in this discipline. "There is a plethora of studies about the way that brain and mind impact the body

Positive people with a positive mental attitude can feel the effect on their health due to a reduced risk of sickness and an overall increase in wellbeing. According to the Mayo Clinic suggests that many advantages to health have been affected by positive attitudes which include a longer life as well as a higher resistance to common cold, lessening the risk of depression, improved heart health, less stress levels, as well as overall mental and physical health.

The current understanding of how positive attitudes affect the health of a person is not clear. One idea, that was discovered through researchers at the Mayo Clinic, is that people who have positive outlooks can better cope with anxiety and stress. Additionally, there is a connection that was observed between people who are positive and those who lead healthy lifestyles by exercising, diet as well as social interaction.

A positive attitude can help one in coping better in the everyday responsibilities of daily life. This brings joy into your everyday life, and helps you keep your mind off of worries and negative thoughts. If you make it your way of living and practice it, you will see positive modifications to your daily life making them better, more cheerful and prosperous. When you have a positive outlook, you are able to see the good aspect of life. You become hopeful and believe that the best is going to come through. This is definitely a state of mind to be developed and strengthened.

Benefits of having an optimistic and positive attitude:

The first and most important thing is Better Health and More energy assists in meeting objectives and achieving success. It also gives you more strength and power within.

I've had patients who suffered from major illness and I advise them that within the next two or three months, they'll be 100% recuperated. Positive people generally recover in this interval or earlier. However, I've also seen patients who were unhappy or unhappy and the time to recover was more lengthy.

I'm sure that you've seen the saying"Live for the present, since yesterday is over and tomorrow will never be here. Live and live the present day like it was the last day of your life.

ONE WAY TO IMPROVE YOUR ATTITUDE IS TO GO OUT AND HELP SOMEONE IN NEED.

Chapter 11: Do Not Be Overweight

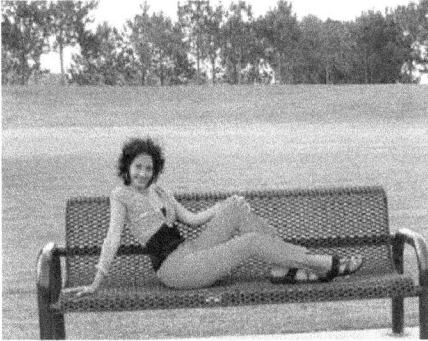

Statistics on obese people within the U.S. vary depending upon whom you speak to, and here are two reliable sources. One source states that 78.3 percent are overweight. including obese (one with more than 20 percent overweight).

* Percentage of adults aged 20 and older that are overweight: 33.9% (2007-2008)

* Percentage of adults aged 20 or over who are obese (and not overweight): 34.4% (2007-2008)

Another source points to the results of the current Gallup Healthways Well-Being index, which indicates that 63.1 percent of adult population within the U.S. were either overweight or obese in 2009.

That means that somewhere between 63 and 78 percent of U.S. Americans are overweight. It's quite a lot, wouldn't suggest?

Every pound more of weight you gain, you cut down your lifespan by a month. Thus, a person who is over 24 pounds would have a shorter lifespan by 2 years. If you're obese it is more likely to be diagnosed with some kinds of cancer. Based on the American Cancer Society (2003) overweight people are more at likelihood of

* Cancer of the breast (after menopausal)

* Cervical cancer

* Retinal or Colon cancer

* Esophageal cancer

. Cancer of the gall bladder

. Kidney cancer

* Cancer of the liver

* Multiple myeloma

* Non-Hodgkin lymphoma

* Ovarian cancer

* Cancer of the pancreas

* Stomach cancer (in men)

* Uterine cancer.

. According to the American Cancer Society (2008) states that 14 to 20 percent of the deaths caused by cancer within the U.S. can be attributed due to weight gain or obesity issues.

The reason most population in the United States have a weight problem is due to the way we eat. Americans consume a lot of processed food containing unneeded calories, chemicals as well as preservatives. They snack on all every moment. More time is spent taking in than removing, and so you carry extra fat.

How Do I Lose Weight?

It requires willpower and determination, with God's assistance to conquer the urge. Like any other problem you'd like to get rid of, it is important to plan your approach to ensure you don't fail. What should I do when that hunger pangs kick in and I'm tempted to consume food? drinking a glass of water will help to ward off hunger pangs. Since

In the event of dehydration, it can trigger cravings for food. It is essential to drink plenty of drinking water throughout the day. It is likely that if you drink the recommended amount of water after meals, you'll be more satisfied, and are less likely to be hungry in between meals.

The ideal food that you can eat for weight loss are healthy natural food items that God has created, and a small number of refined and processed foods, which are usually very calorific. This is a good example that will provide you with an idea. Whole baked potatoes contain approximately. 100 calories. It is a natural food and not processed. Potato chips, which have been made with refined oils do not come from nature and the potato chips contain 10 calories! Which is going to fill you more quickly, the whole baked potato or 10 chips of potato, because both have 100 calories?

Chapter 12: Avoid Radiation

Cell phones Radiation from phones may be a cause of cancer, according to the World Health Organization. It has now put cell phone usage in the exact "carcinogenic hazard" category as the exhaust of engines, lead and chloroform. The team, comprised of 31 researchers from 14 nations, which includes those from the United States, made the choice after examining peer-reviewed research regarding the safety of cell phones. The researchers found evidence to label the exposure of individuals to cell phones as "possibly carcinogenic to humans."

Mobile phones emit radiofrequency energy which is a type of non-ionizing electromagnetic radiation that may be absorbed by tissue close to the area the location where the phone is. The quantity of radiofrequency energy the user exposed to will depend on the type of technology used by the phone, as well as the distance between its antenna and the phone user in addition to the amount and frequency of usage, as well as the users distance to cell towers. Some case-control studies in Sweden found

Significantly statistically-significant trends in the increase of risk of brain cancer in relation to the overall amount of mobile phone usage and time of usage among those who first started using phones before the age of 20. Hardell L, Carlberg M Hansson Mild K. Pooled analysis of study-control cases on brain malignant tumors as well as the utilization of cell and mobile phones that include deceased and living participants. International Journal of Oncology 2011; 38(5):1465-1474. [PubMed Abstract]

The results of the biggest international study of cell phones and cancer were revealed in the year the year 2010. The study showed that participants of the study who were using cell phones for a period of 10 years or longer have doubled their risk of brain glioma. It is a form of tumor.

What Should One Do Then?

It is best not to own one. I myself have given up mine, and am grateful for it. However, if you are unable to survive without one, I suggest using these tips. You should reserve the use of mobile phones to have shorter conversations, or when the landline isn't accessible.

Make use of a device that is hands-free with a greater distance between the mobile as well as the face of the person using it.

Hands-free devices reduce the radiofrequency radiation that is absorbed by the head due to the fact that the antenna, the main source of energy isn't positioned against the head.

Wi-Fi

Wireless Internet routers and Wi-Fi devices utilize dangerous electromagnetic radiation EMFs, to transmit their signals to computers. If you've got a Wi-Fi Internet router in your workplace or at home there is a huge EMF exposure all every day, even if your computer is off. The amount of radiation that is thought of by scientists as well as health professionals as being potentially harmful. It is recommended that you turn off your Wi-Fi off, and to use directly connected cables.

The main reason for this data to come to the public's attention is that a lot of schools currently within the U.S. have WiFi and certain students attending these schools have chest pains, headaches breathing issues, headaches, etc. while at school. But these issues disappear when they are off the campus. In the U.S. the schools are not taking action to address this issue and the majority of parents have to the children in the grip of

MICROWAVE FOOD IS DANGEROUS TO EAT

Microwave ovens can be found throughout the majority of American households. They provide a speedy method to cook and heat food items, making them ideal in today's hectic world however, they are harmful to your well-being ! Indeed microwaves are now common in American homes, and they have been replaced by the traditional oven and stovetop to cook food. Russians have been able to ban the use of microwaves due its negative effects on health. The impacts that Russian researchers observed were the development of cancer-causing agents and increased risk for cancer-related development and reduced nutritional value of foods.

Prior to WWII (1939-45) it's been recognized that microwaves are dangerous to our biological systems. Food items that were prepared, heated, or defrosted within the microwave oven resulted in substantial changes to the blood of those who were tested. The changes were characterized by a decrease of hemoglobin concentrations in general as well as

cholesterol levels, particularly those of HDL cholesterol levels, particularly HDL LDL. Lymphocytes (which comprise white blood cells),

The results showed a distinct reduction in short-term time after the consumption of food items from microwave ovens than consumption of any other types.

The study found a significant connection between the quantity of microwave energy present in the irradiated foods and the luminescence of luminescent bacteria that were exposed to blood samples from people who consumed the food. The result is that the energy of technology like microwave energy can be transferred into the human body inductively through radiation foods. The process relies on the physical principle and has already been established in research. The results of the microwave irradiated foods on human in contrast to unirradiated foods, reveal variations in blood levels of the test subjects that indicate an early pathogenicity like the beginning of cancer.

Chapter 13: Take No Supplements

April 13, 2011more than one-half of U.S adults consume supplementation to their diets, according to the CDC, Centers for Disease Control.

The report, that is part of the Data Brief of the CDC's National Center for Health Statistics' Data Brief, looked at the use of dietary supplements among adult adults in the period 2003-2006 in comparison with the use of supplements in 1988 and 1994.

"Dietary supplement use has increased in adults over age 20 since 1994, and we have over one-half of Americans taking one or more supplements a day," declares research author Jaime Gahche, MPH, Nutrition epidemiologist with the National Center for Health Statistics located in Bethesda, Md.

Supplements for mineral and vitamin intake necessary in your diet? What kinds are necessary and how much of them should be consumed? Answering these questions is easy If God had wanted us to consume supplements, such as Vitamin C then He would have created a tree which produces Vitamin C tablets. Instead, He created a variety of fruit trees. Each fruits contain the Vitamin C the body needs. The American population has been taught that vitamins are essential to their overall health. The actual requirement for minerals and vitamins has been significantly exaggerated. The quantity of nutrients the human body requires over the course of a year is tiny. Each vitamin is a good one.

minerals that the body needs is found in food we consume.

It is commonplace to eat them by the bucketful with great cost, but there's no proof that vitamins do us benefit, and may even harm us according to research conducted by scientists. As a attack on the multimillion-dollar food supplement industry, a analysis of 67 trials of vitamins has revealed that, far from extending lives, they can in fact cut it down.

There's "no convincing evidence" that antioxidants reduce the chance of premature death, and certain of them can increase the likelihood of premature death as per the study that was published by The Cochrane Collaboration. Goran Bjelakovich, the visiting researcher in charge of the systematic review conducted at Copenhagen University, said: "We could find no evidence to support taking antioxidant supplements to reduce the risk of dying earlier in healthy people or patients with various diseases."

"The research findings suggest that more likely, individuals with beta-carotene in their trial groups Vitamin A, beta-carotene as well as vitamin E, had increased levels of mortality. Researchers separated the 47 trials that had the lowest risk of bias, and they observed a significant increase in deaths rate. If taken in isolation Vitamin A was linked with a 16 per cent increase in death rate, beta-carotene was associated with 7 percent increase and vitamin E was associated with a four percentage rise.

In a piece in The Health Reporter by Robert McCarter Doctor of Philosophy, these supplements don't have the properties meant for humans. When it comes to extraction and fragmentation of elements, the nutrients are useless after being removed.

Vitamins isolated lose their effectiveness. There is technology that allows the creation of the grain of wheat the lab.

All the chemical components that are required may be replicated, and transformed into a grain of whey However, when it's dumped in the soil, it won't grow. Why? because the wheat grain isn't natural.

Man can't improve on the way that our Creator gave us to obtain the vitamins and minerals we need. As an example, there are numerous warnings about using Vitamin C. There are adverse consequences. Vitamin C contains an anti-vitamin D impact. It means that when you supplement with Vitamin C the body will require more Vitamin D. The other negative side effect could be Vitamin C can also reduce the supply of B Vitamins especially B6 and B12. A single orange contains 70 milligrams Vitamin C and has .11 milligrams of thiamine .05 milligrams riboflavin etc...The orange is also rich in minerals, including 52 milligrams calcium, 18 milligrams phosphorus, etc. .... If you choose to take the Vitamin C supplement, instead of eating the entire orange God made, you're damaging your body since you're not getting the full amount of Vitamin C and minerals and so on. in the fruit.

"NATURAL VERSUS SYNTHETIC VITAMINS

Paul Stitt, a biochemist as well as food scientist at several of the biggest corporations within the United States, reports that the government has regulations that require only 3 percent of nutritional supplement must be made up of natural ingredients before it can be identified as "natural" He points out the fact that synthetic vitamins can be so harmful, they must be removed.

cheaper, and more affordable, and it's likely that the majority are less expensive, and a lot of "natural" vitamins on the market today are 97 percent synthesized.

According to him, it will take 30 oranges in order to make one 1,000 mg. vitamin C tablet and a bottle of pure vitamin C tablets would cost around 4 hundred dollars. Be aware, though, that even if the bottles of Vitamin C was made entirely of oranges, and the price was around four hundred dollars, it will not be organic Vitamin C because it is separated from the fruit and is not containing the fiber, phytochemicals, different vitamins, enzymes and so on. Therefore, it is best to obtain the Vitamin C by sourcing it from its original origin, which is the food itself.

Chapter 14: Prescribed Drugs Can Cause Cancer

DANGERS OF PRESCRIBED DRUGS

The numbers are difficult to believe! Every year, around 2.2 millions US hospital patients are affected by adverse drug reaction (ADRs) in response to prescription medications.Of the 783,936 deaths each year from medical malpractices that occur in the normal course of medicine around 106,000 of them are due to prescription medications, as reported by the Death by Medicine. This is also a moderate amount. According to some experts, it ought to be higher than 200,000 due to the number there are a lot of cases that have not been reported of drug-related adverse reactions.

"Another JAMA article ("Incidence of adverse drug reactions among the hospitalized patient," 1998 1200-1205). 1200-1205) revealed that 20% of new medications contain serious side effects that are not known (on to the well-known effects). Over

100,000 Americans each year die due to being on the right track with their prescribed medication! Be aware, however that this is not an admission from inside the medical system. There is a chance that the real scenario is even more dire?

The number of people who die from prescription medications each year than through car crashes within the U.S. ! !!! !

I WANT TO SHARE WITH YOU THE SIDE

EFFECTS OF JUST TWO DIFFERENT

PRESCRIBED DRUGS, FOSAMAX and CHEMOTHERAPY

FOSAMAX

For instance, bisphosphonates are the most frequently prescribed osteoporosis medications like Fosamax, Boniva, Actonel and Reclast and others. They come with a long list of potential side consequences. If you'd like to find out about the negative effects of the medication that you're taking, search on Google and type into side effects for the medication you're using. For example, Fosamax, here are the adverse effects that are described by google.

Side Effects of Fosamax - for the Consumer

Fosamax

Each medicine has its own potential unwanted side negative effects . Consult your physician for any of the following common side effects continue or get worse when taking Fosamax

Diarrhea, constipation; nausea and feeling full or bloated Flu-like symptoms that occur when treatment begins nausea; headache; slight back, muscle or joint pain; slight stomach upset or pain nausea, changes in taste and vomiting.

Take immediate medical care If any of these severe negative side effects happen while taking Fosamax:

difficult breathing; tightness of the chest, swelling of the face, mouth and throat or tongue) or Black, tarry, or bloody stomach pains bleeding or coughing blood and painful or difficult swallowing; mouth sores the appearance of a new or worsening constant heartburn; red inflamed, blistered or peeling skin muscles, bone or joint discomfort (especially in the hip area, thigh, or groin) as well as persistent or extreme stomach or sore throat and swelling of legs, hands joints, or hands and pain or swelling in the jaw. Signs of the presence of low blood calcium (for example , spasms, tightness, or twitches in the muscles of your body; numbness or tingling sensations in your hands, feet or in the mouth).

This isn't an exhaustive description of all the side effects which could happen. If you are concerned regarding side effects, consult your doctor. Consult your physician to get medical advice on the consequences . In addition to this lengthy list of adverse consequences that may occur shortly following the start of treatment it has only been recently that the emergence of new, longer-lasting side effects that are more hazardous are being identified including an increase in the possibility of cancer in the esophagus, unusual femur fractures, as well as kidney insufficiency.

CHEMOTHERAPY

SIDE EFFECTS OF CHEMOTHERAPY FOR TREATING CANCER

One of the most hazardous substances that we can take into our bodies are those which are used in the fight against cancer.

Thirteen drugs are used in chemotherapy and their consequent side effects (as listed in the drugs package inserts for physicians), which include: destruction of the immune system, leukopenia, hemorrhage, gonadal suppression, bone marrow depression, phlebosclerosis (hardening of the veins), severe cellulites, vesication(blistering), tissue necrosis(death), fever, chills, nausea, prolonged vomiting, partial or total hair loss, lethargy, disorientation, ataxis(inability to coordinate muscle movements), dysarthria(impaired speech), anorexia, entertitis, stomatitis, erythema, (morbid redness of the skin), anemia, liver failure, kidney failure, CANCER and death. It is true that chemotherapy causes cancer, so why should someone take chemotherapy in order to treat cancer?

FOOD INSTEAD OF DRUGS CAN BE OUR MEDICINE

In 1995 in 1995, in 1995, Dr. Richard Besser of the federal Centers for Disease Control and Prevention (CDC) calculated the amount of unneeded antibiotics prescribed each year in viral diseases to be around 20 million. in 2003 the Besser estimated the number to be 20 million. Besser spoke in terms of 10 million unneeded antibiotics that are prescribed each year. But what exactly are the best natural antibiotics?

RAW GARLIC IS A NATURAL ANTIBIOTIC

The antibiotics that are prescribed to you be used to kill bacteria. They cannot eradicate viruses. They also have numerous negative side negative effects. Garlic (MUST MUST BE AWARE) does not only kill bacteria, but also viruses. It does not cause any adverse side effects.

Except for the scent. One way that I've had my patients take their garlic under control is to place a cup of lemon juice into a blender, along with 2 or 3 cloves of garlic, and blend. Strain it, and consume it. It is recommended to drink it along with your dinner so that it isn't excessively strong for your stomach. It is also possible to use other juices, such as citrus juices, tomato juice and so on. You can also include a teaspoon of sea salt to taste if you want.

Garlic is also a source of sulfur compounds that may help boost the immune system's natural defenses to fight cancer and also can help to slow down cancer growth.

Chapter 15: Chemicals Found In Many Products Can Cause Cancer

It's not possible to go through all products or substances with these ingredients in this post. I will only cover only a handful of them to show the importance of reading the list of ingredients in products we utilize.

Choose clothes that do not require being dry cleaned. A lot of dry cleaners make use of a chemical called perchloroethylene. This chemical has been proven to cause liver and kidney injury and tumors in animals exposed repeatedly to the chemical to it through breathing. purchasing clothes that do not need dry-cleaning, or even washing them by yourself will minimize the exposure to the chemical. If you need to dry clean your clothes, pull them out of their plastic bag and let them air outdoors or in a different space prior to wearing.

Did you take the time to looked up the ingredients on your shaving cream, child's bubble baths, mouthwash, and have you seen mouthwash and noticed the "warning label" on your toothpaste box? ?

Why are toothpastes labelled with an indication such as

Warning labels: Keep it away from children younger than 6 years old. Don't ingest. ... If you accidentally inhale Seek professional help or call an emergency poison control centre immediately.

The warnings on the product are there to provide a reason. It's a fact several manufacturers utilize certain untested and controversial chemicals primarily due to their low cost and also give the illusion of functioning properly. However, more important for manufacturers is that they are very inexpensive to refill the bottle, which means they generate a higher revenue margin. However, the residues of over 400 chemicals that are toxic are detected in blood of human beings as well as fat tissue.

Did you KNOW that KIDS Bubble baths come with warning labels? Why? The reason is that the sodium lauryl sulfate present in them is a bactericide that eats from the mucous lining the skin, causing urinary tract infections that are bad for girls who are of any vârstă. A world-renowned expert in toxicology, toxicologist and Chairman of the

Nationwide Cancer Prevention Coalition, and co-author of Safe Shopping's Bible Dr. Samuel Epstein has said that "Lifelong use of these products... clearly poses major avoidable cancer risks to the great majority of the U.S. consumers, particularly in infants and young children."

USE NO SUNSCREENS

Skin cancer is one of the most often diagnosed cancer for females and males. There are more than a million cases identified each year, and the number of people in their 20s having skin cancer than before. The sun's harmful rays cause skin cancer. It is recommended keep away from the sunlight.

Studies have proven that all of us require 10-15 minutes of sunlight direct on our bodies at least 5 each week. Sunlight provides the actual Vitamin D instead of synthetic Vitamin D which is in our food which can harm our body. Sunlight is an effective regulater of a variety of the body's functions. We all NEED THE SUNSHINE. However, excessive exposure to anything could cause harm to us, and this includes the sun's rays. It is not recommended to use sunlamps because they are associated with skin cancer.

Nothing can rival the natural sunlight that God has provided us with. If one sunbathes, one should avoid using any kind of sunscreen or oils-based lotions on the skin.

There are two major reason why sunscreen causes cancer. The first, and the most important using sunscreen prevents the skin from taking in the UV rays of the sun. This is what sunscreens are supposed to perform, right? However, when it does this it blocks the production of vital vitamin D, a essential nutrient our bodies requires to fight off up to 25 chronic illnesses. In particular, prostate cancer osteoporosis, breast cancer the heart and schizophrenia.

The reality is that the majority of people who live in the Northern Hemisphere have a chronic deficit with vitamin D. Wearing sunscreen, they're stripping their bodies of possibly the most essential vitamin they'll ever need to be well.

The other reason sunscreen causes cancer is that it's made up of harmful chemicals that are that are in the form of synthetic scent, chemical colors and petroleum-based products that are that are used to stabilize and fillers. The chemicals get absorbed by the skin, where they

get into the bloodstream, and cause destruction in the body's immune system. The artificial fragrances, by their own, can contain hundreds of carconigenic chemicals which harm the heart, liver and or even cause tumors of the body.

The world is now spending billions in sun-blockers seeking to shield their bodies from harm that doesn't pose a risk in any way: of 300 sunbathers, 299 don't develop skin cancer. If sun exposure causes skin cancer, why is it that the skin cancers usually appear around the areas of your body that are not subject to sunlight?

The evidence from interviews and documentation has shown that the FDA knew about the dangers of sun blockers more than a decade, without informing to the general public.

I'm hoping I've informed you of the fact that it is important to know the ingredients (chemicals such as chemicals.) which are present in the products we purchase to determine if they be more harmful than beneficial for your overall health.

Chapter 16: Practicing Safe Sex

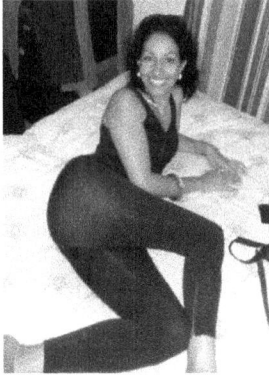

It is best to avoid sexual assault by with only one person - someone that isn't suffering from an STI and who has sexual relations only with you. That's what I strongly suggest. A partner you truly love and a love for your partner is exactly what God had in mind from the start. It is not just about keeping your body healthy, but also spiritually and mentally.

If you have multiple sexual partners, here is what I suggest: always wear condoms or alternative methods to prevent contraception.

They play a role in the development of specific cancers. They are generally sexually passed. The human papillomavirus (HPV) is a factor in numerous cases of cervical cancer as well as increasing the chance of developing cancers in other areas including cervical cancers of the head and neck, anal cancers, and tumors of the vulva and penis. Hepatitis B or C may increase the chance for liver cancer.

The changes you make don't mean that you won't develop cancer, but it does lower the risk of it.

Chapter 17: Get Antioxidants

Cancer is now a common occurrence throughout our lives due to numerous reasons. Mayo clinic confirms that inadvertent eating habits, excess weight smoking, exposure to contaminants and some microorganisms are the most significant factors that cause cancer.

Genetic causes are also an important factor in the development of certain forms of cancer. Likewise, exposure to ultraviolet rays of the sun is the main cause for skin cancer.

Lutein as well as Zeanthin are two antioxidants that come from cruciferous veggies like cabbage, Brussels sprouts, broccoli and the kale. Both antioxidants have potent properties for fighting cancer of the prostate. Many fruits and veggies contain antioxidants as well as minerals and vitamins that can be extremely beneficial for the prevention and treatment of various cancers.

Fruits like papayas, citrus and a lot of veggies are loaded with ascorbic acid. It is an antioxidant that helps boost the immune system in fighting cancerous cells. Fruits are full of nutrients and minerals which aid in stopping cancerous cells from growing and help to protect the body. Peas, walnuts and almost all other nuts are abundant in antioxidants, which slow the growth of cancer cells.

Teas have also cancer fighting characteristics, and green tea in particular has a lot of cancer-fighting power. Since green teas originate created from tea leaves unfermented they have a large amount of antioxidants often referred to polyphenols.

Polyphenols fight free radicals that are the main reason for most illnesses and cancerous cell growth. Polyphenols fight free radicals and help protect healthy cells throughout the body. Garlic and onions have allium compounds which aid in the development of in strengthening our immune system. Ginger and turmeric can stop cancer cell growth and jalapenos and chili peppers contain capsaicin which helps fight cancer.

Carrots are brimming with of beta-carotene. A high percentage of beta-carotene can be behind the bright orange hue and helps the immune system in preventing certain types of cancer. Research has proven that eating food high in beta-carotene reduces the chance of developing prostate, breast and stomach cancer by 26%.

The majority of cancer-fighting foods contain phytochemicals sometimes referred to as phytonutrient. Over 4,000 phytochemicals are present which are being studied and investigated. The phytonutrients include chemical compounds in plants to prevent illnesses like cancer and the growth of cancerous tumors. There isn't a superfood which contains the full spectrum of phytonutrients. However, having many colors can provide the highest amount of our diets that are that is rich in vegetables and fruits

Mackerel, anchovies and salmon are high of vitamin B and potassium, and omega-3 fats. Consuming a diet that is rich in freshwater fish lowers the chance of developing colorectal cancer by 53%.

The fiber in lentils is high, which can lower the chance of developing cancer. The results of studies have proven that intake of legumes, such as beans, lentils, and peas decrease the chance of developing colorectal cancer and bean fiber also reduces the likelihood of breast cancer. Fiber-rich diets reduce the likelihood of breast cancer development by 20% when compared with those who don't have that consumption.

Chapter 18: Fiber And Cancer

High fiber foods are essential for healthy well-being, and the evidence to support the necessity of regular fiber intake is overwhelming. fruit, vegetables, and whole grains are among the most important. The consumption of high fiber foods reduces the amount of cholesterol and keeps the levels within a certain range. It helps prevent digestive diseases such as diverticulitis.

White rice, processed food items as well as white bread and all grain products contain fiber in their entirety. It's a bit scholarly from an nutrient standpoint because bran, germ, and starchy endosperm have their nutrition. Certain people think that the process of processing whole grains in order to make refined grains leads to a decrease of nutritional value. However, it isn't true. In order to make up for diminished food value that is lost during processing it is recommended that the fine grain flours to be improved, and a few artificial vitamins and minerals are incorporated, but this is not able to restore the loss of nutritional value.

The wheat grain contains minerals such as calcium, magnesium and copper. It also contains iron, zinc, sodium and manganese. Vitamins that are present include thiamin and niacin, Vitamin C, pantothenic acid folate vitamin B6 as well as Vitamin E. The majority of carbohydrate molecules are broken down into glucose. However, processed grains can be metabolized faster than whole grains. This rapid metabolism of carbohydrates triggers an increase in blood sugar that can result in a rise in tension hormones and hunger which can cause arteriosclerosis.

Oats, brown rice, millet, barley and whole wheat bread, and rye are all the examples of whole grain. They can take longer time to cook than refined grains, however they're worth it.

Whole grains are a cancer-risk food.

A diet that is rich in whole grain lowers the chance of developing colon cancer. Whole grain food items are made composed of all seeds from cereal plants. The processed grains are stripped of a portion of the grain. It is white grains are found in white pasta and rice. The part that is removed is more healthy and contains a greater amount of fiber over the white portion.

Wholegrains are composed from three components comprising the bran, endosperm and the germ. The germ and bran have a greater proportion of fiber, vitamins and minerals found in the grain. Taking out the bran and germ causes one losing the most nutritious.

The fiber in the body and its cancer-risk.

It is a type of carbohydrate which cannot be digested easily. It passes through the gut as well as into the bowel. It is mostly available in plant-based foods like whole cereals, grains fruit, legumes and legumes (lentils and beans) and even vegetables.

Based on research that has shown whole grain fiber can be more effective in cutting down the risk of getting cancer than the different sources mentioned earlier. To get the best results, consume different sources of fiber such as those listed above.

Change the traditional foods such as pasta, rice biscuits, pasta and bread by eating whole grains like bran, whole wheat cereals, porridge and oats. Every meal, eat the fruits and vegetables you like, but most importantly, fresh.

Tinned and frozen alternatives may be useful if they do not have any preservatives. In order to get the maximum benefit of the fiber content found in vegetable sources, you should eat the outer layer of vegetables such as carrots and potatoes. It is possible to use pulses for beans or lentils in substitute for meat. It is also possible to consume high-fiber snacks like fruits, nuts or plain popcorn seeds and Whole wheat crunchers.

Dieticians advise that adults consume 30g of fiber per day. It could mean taking in more whole grain products such as wholegrain grains (12-24.5g of fiber) whole breakfast toast (8g of fiber) Whole gluten-free pasta made from wheat (5g in fiber)

When purchasing food items make sure you look for "Whole" before the name of the ingredient or item. Oats and brown rice are both whole grains. Wholegrains contain more fibre content than refined items.

What is the role of fiber in reducing the chance of developing cancer in bowels.

Chapter 19: Toxins, Preservatives And Other Chemicals

Pollutants, toxicants and preservatives can be found in us every day via our food and our drinking water and the products we use for cosmetics, such as dirt as well as insecticides and disinfectants.

Phenol, which is a potentially harmful toxin that is found used in the manufacture of air fresheners, disinfectants as well as products to treat bacterial infections. Exposure to phenol over time and other toxins has a harmful effect on the nerve and respiratory systems of our bodies. They are also responsible for the development of cancer and other ailments.

The importance of education is in the dangers for these substances to individual so that you may minimize the danger and exposure. Once you have been educated about the effects of chemicals and the toxins listed on the labels of products You will be able to make an educated choices and opt for non-toxic alternatives.

Below is a list of harmful substances as well as products that they can be present.

1 Azodicarbonamide

The material is used in flip-flops as well as spongy plastic items. This may appear harmless since bread makers employ it in the production of more supple and attractive breads, however it is the World Health Organization (WHO) has pointed it out in the increasing cases of respiratory problems as well as skin irritations after frequent exposure.

2 Dioxane.

This chemical is used in dyes for shampoos Deodorants, cosmetics, as well as food supplements. The chemical is associated with cases of eye, nose or throat irritation. It's a well-known source of kidney and liver destruction.

3 Phthalates

These chemicals are commonly found in the form of perfumes, hairsprays nail polishes, cosmetic products Shower curtains, food packaging and other plastic items. Consuming or swallowing them, as well as contact with products containing phthalates can impact the reproductive system of humans or can cause cancer.

4 Lead

The lead in the environment is poisonous to your body and it has been linked to problems with the brain, miscarriage hearing loss, and kidney damage. It can be found in the old paints and drinking water.

5.BPA

Bisphenol A is also called BPA is banned from infant and child products following its connection to cancers, birth defects and reproductive toxicity. However, it is still found in food products such as canned drinks.

6 Fire retardants

They are typically present in furniture, to decrease the risk of fire from cigarettes stubs. The use of flame retardants has been linked with the increase of cancer risk, hyperactivity, and lower IQ

7 Arsenic

Arsenic is an extremely deadly poison for rats, however it can be discovered in seafood like oysters, mussels, clams as well as in drinking water too. A small amount of it could cause bladder, lung, skin cancer or hormone imbalance.

8 Triclosan

This ingredient is present in soaps and toothpaste. While it's not allowed by the FDA for soaps, it's still utilized as an antimicrobial and is also used in toothpastes. When it is accumulated within the toothbrush, it could get into the circulation system, causing stomach and hormone problems.

9 Perfluorinated Chemicals (PFCs)

PFCs can be found in everyday home products like carpets, cookware mattress, bedding, containers for food and beverages. PFCs are harmful and could result in ADHD as well as alter TSH levels. Studies on animals have revealed that it can adversely impact the liver and can cause difficulties with the development of fetuses.

10 Mercury

It is typically found in seafood, shellfish as well as household items like lamps, cosmetics, thermometers and batteries. The presence of high levels of mercury within the body could cause problems with development in fetuses.

11. Atrazine

It is a herbicide that is used for crops. It can be used in water that is filtered for drinking. It has been associated with reproductive defects, and hormonal disruptions. To be safe, choose organic ingredients and an water purifier to remove the chemicals.

12. Toluene

The chemical is commonly found in candle scents. The study conducted at South Carolina University reveals that burning candles that are scented emit alkenes, alkanes and toluene. These can put your health in danger. The frequent use of candles with scented scents could lead to health risks such as allergies, cancer, asthma, and many other illnesses.

13 PFSAS

These are known as Polyfluoroalkyl Substances (PFSAS) These are substances found in plastic bags. If you frequently microwave popcorn then the PFSAS gets into the popcorn once consumed, it may adversely impact the immune system and cause liver or kidney toxicity, and newborn weight gain.

14 Volatile Organic Compounds (VOCs)

They are harmful chemicals used in cleaning materials that can trigger headaches as well as eye, throat and nasal irritation. These chemicals can cause cancer as well. Aerosols, detergents and cleansers made from natural compounds must be taken into consideration.

15 Dioxins

They are present in meat products from animals milk fish, shellfish. This can negatively impact the hormones in your body, as well as fertility health, and can increase the risk of developing cancer.

16 Polytetrafluoroethylene (PTFE)

The PTFE compound is an excellent chemical that is found in cookware. If you cookware is overheated this can trigger the symptoms of flu, along with other respiratory issues, or possibly cancer.

17. Formaldehyde

Formaldehyde is one of the chemicals used in air fresheners, soaps, cosmetics cleaning products, soaps and lotions. This chemical is the ingredient employed in embalming. It's extremely toxic and can be flammable even at temperatures of room temperature. Exposure to it repeatedly can lead to cancer.

18. DEET

DEET is found in insect repellents, liquid sprays stick and lotions. exposure in large quantities can cause skin irritation, rash blisters, redness and swellings. Ingestion of DEET can cause an omission, stomach upset that is severe nausea and stomach upset. The drug has been linked to seizures.

19. Perchlorate

It's a chemical component that is used in the manufacture of rocket fuel, as well as fireworks. It's also in drinking water and milk. Research has shown that exposure to it for long periods has caused thyroid cancer as well as the balance of thyroid hormones in rodents. Balance of thyroid hormones regulates metabolism, brain and organ growth in infants.

20, Aluminum

Aluminum can be found in containers as well as pans and sheets. It's used in the production of colorants and flours Exposure in high doses are believed to be the cause of Alzheimer's disease and the brain to damage for those suffering from kidney disease.

21. Nonylphenols

Nonylphenols can be found in laundry soaps, personal care items and other detergents. It is detected in the milk that lactating mothers give their babies, their blood and urine. It's been demonstrated to be a cause of developmental issues in mice and rats.

22. Polybrominated Diphenyl Ethers

Polybrominated Diphenyl Ethers known as PBDE is used to serve for their role as flame-resistants on mattresses and cushions. The chemical causes neurological problems for humans. As you will spend about more than a third of your time in the night, it's important to choose a safe and non-toxic alternative, even though it is pricier.

23. Chloroform

Chloroform can be released into the air through the chlorination process for water used to drink, pools and waste. The inhalation of chloroform can trigger liver issues depression, cancer, and liver issues.

24. Silica:

Silica is an anti-caking agent as well as an ingredient in food products. It regulates thickness. It is employed as a dough-modifying agent and an anti-foaming ingredient, and also in pharmaceuticals for excipients. Silica particles when caught within the lung tissues, result in scarring and inflammation. They reduce the capacity of the lungs to breathe, which can cause permanent injury, and in certain cases, cause lung cancer.

What can you do to stay clear of poisonous toxins?

1 Limit the amount mercury you inhale by choosing your fish carefully

2. Reduce the amount of bluefish, tuna as well as shark and swordfish rather, purchase wild salmon Pacific cod, also known as tilapia or

3 Don't eat fried items Grill, broil or bake your food.

4. Purchase organic vegetables and fruits

5. Filter your water to avoid heavy metals from your drinking water.

6. Limit the usage of Teflon or any other pan that has a non-stick coating. Use stainless steel instead as well as cast iron cookware.

7. Do not microwave inside plastic products and only use packaging that bears the "Microwave-safe" label or ceramic containers.

8. Avoid the usage of soaps that are antibacterial because They may be contaminated with pesticides and may be absorbed into skin. Soap that is normal for 20 seconds can be as efficient.

9. Reduce the usage of herbicides as well as pesticides because toxic substances can be absorbed via the skin, or by inhalation

10. Take off your shoes prior to stepping into the house, as there are dust can cause toxins, and it is possible to enter your home with shoes in place for a long time.

11. Reduce the usage of bleach. Instead, try lemon juice instead for whitening.

12. Check the ingredients of personal care items

13. Beware of chemical contact to your clothing, particularly the softeners you use in your dryer or washer.

14. Cleansers from professional brands are best left outside for at least 7 hours to keep chemical odors and chemicals from coming back into your home

15. Clean your home with filters. Make use of an HEPA filter since it is able to trap tiny particles.

16. Make sure to use only products for personal care made by companies who don't employ substances that are toxic in their manufacturing procedure.

Chapter 20: Stop Smoking

The damage caused by smoking cigarettes affects every organ of the body. The research has shown that more than 16 million Americans suffer from diseases that are caused by smoking cigarettes. Every time a person dies from tobacco it is estimated that there are thirty people who suffer from ailments that are caused by smoking. Smoking tobacco is a leading reason for heart disease, diabetes lung conditions, and chronic obstructive pulmonary disorder (COPD) which is a chronic bronchitis as well as Emphysema. Smoking raises the risk of various eye diseases such as tuberculosis, arthritis, rheumatoid and other immune system related issues.

Smoking secondhand is the cause of more than 40,000 deaths in non-smokers as well as the deaths of 400 babies every year. Smoking secondhand can cause lung cancer, strokes, as well as coronary heart diseases. The children exposed increase the risk of sudden infant death syndrome middle ear diseases as well as acute respiratory infections asthma, and slowed lung growth.

Smoking cigarettes contains a variety of harmful substances that can be harmful for smokers as well as non-smokers. Smoking even a small amount is extremely damaging for your body. Out of the more than 7,000 chemicals found in cigarettes, around 250 are highly dangerous. This list includes ammonia, hydrogen cyanide carbon monoxide. The 69 harmful chemical compounds in cigarettes could cause cancer. Carcinogenic chemicals include:

Aromatic amino amines

Specific to tobacco nitrosamines

Benzene

Beryllium (a poisonous metal)

Acetaldehyde

Cumene

Arsenic

1,3-Butadiene (a hazardous gas)

Chromium (a metal element)

Vinyl chloride

Ethylene oxide

The polycyclic aromatic hydrocarbons (PAHs)

Nickel (a metal element)

Polonium-210 (a radioactive chemical element)

Cadmium (a poisonous metal)

Formaldehyde

Smoking and Cancer Risk:

Smoking tobacco is the reason for 20 percent of cancers, and 30percent to deaths throughout the United States. The majority of lung cancers as well as lung cancer related deaths stem from smoking cigarettes.

Smoking raises the risk for different cancers.

Esophagus

Liver

Cervix

Pancreas

Stomach

Bladder

Mouth

Colon/rectum

Kidney

The acute myeloid leukemia.

Pharynx (throat)

Larynx (voice box)

Pipes, cigarettes and cigarettes cause cancer. There's no way to make a safe use of tobacco that isn't associated with the possibility of getting cancer.

10 methods to quit smoking

1. Avoid situations that can trigger cravings for smoking.

Find out what triggers an urge to smoke. These could be people, places or events or stress, food and maybe even foods you were enjoying as a hobby together with cigarettes. Be aware of your choices and avoid setting yourself up for a rebound. If you were smoking while speaking via the phone, try to keep engaged instead of smoking.

2. Consider nicotine rehabilitation.

Talk to your doctor for a prescription medication that is non-nicotine-free to stop smoking. You can also use quick-acting nicotine treatment options such as gum or nasal sprays, inhalers, and gums; they can aid in overcoming excessive cravings. If you combine them together with nicotine patches that are long-acting. Electronic cigarettes aren't any better than nicotine replacement medications.

3. Relaxation techniques

Smoking cigarettes was one of your methods to manage anxiety, battling the urges by itself is exhausting. Consider deep breathing, visualization massage, relaxation of the muscles as well as listening to music that is soft and even yoga.

4. Chew gum

Chew sugar-free gum or carrots, nuts, candy, seeds or other healthy snacks or substitute.

5. Physical exercise

Exercise can help you curb the craving for tobacco. In a brief burst of disorienting activities, such as walking or running can make all the differences.

6. Deferment.

Stop the urge to smoke by engaging in other things to do. You can give yourself 10, 20 30, 40 50, 60 or even more time. The time will arrive when you'll be staying for indefinitely for weeks, days and months before breaking your addiction.

7. Peer influence.

Find a group of people who will help you to overcome the addiction to tobacco. Talk to each other, have some laughs with people who share your interests Contact support or advice from experts who have an established track record of results, and then spend some your time enjoying loved ones and family members who mean the world to you.

8. Do not take "just one last drink"

Don't believe that you'll take just one last beverage as it is likely to smoke again. Don't drink an extra drink when you are at the house or with your family as the likelihood is that you'll continue this drinking habit.

9. Positive self-talk.

Call yourself your own name, to remind yourself that it is beneficial to quit smoking tobacco. For example:

Becoming better

Helping to protect your loved ones from the hazards from secondhand smoke as described in the previous paragraphs.

Money to save

Feeling better

The more you succeed in resisting the urge to smoke the closer you will be toward stopping smoking cigarettes.

Chapter 21: Lycopene

Lycopene is a natural substance found in carotenoids such as carrots, oranges and sweet potatoes. The fruits that have red, yellow and orange coloration are abundant in lycopene. Studies have shown that lycopene ranks one of the three most popular carotenoids in addition to alpha-carotene and beta-carotene.

What is the best way to utilize Lycopene supplements?

Lycopene blocks the growth of cancerous tumors. Carotenoids typically slow down the growth of cancerous cells as well as encourage the development of normal cells. Consuming a wide range of carotenoids can result in an efficient result since Lycopene isn't a single ingredient.

Carotenoids help prevent the growth of plaque (arteriosclerosis) within blood vessels. In preventing the hardening process of fat, carotenoids shield the blood vessels in the arterial.

The immune system of your body functions better thanks to the antioxidants found in carotenoids, which help combat diseases and infections. The consumption of carotene rich foods boosts the number of mononuclear cells. They are essential to the immunity's bodily functions. Carotenoids boost levels of the interleukin which is a by-product from the white blood cell. they play a significant role in the immune system's function.

Zeaxanthin as well as leutien, are both carotenoids found in the macular tissues in the eyeball. They filter out the damaging sunlight's ultraviolet rays and stop them from damaging the retina.

As we get older as we age, it's important to consume food sources of carotenoids in order in order to stop macular degeneration. Lycopene from tomatoes can prevent prostate cancer and enlargement. Recent research has shown that the preparation of tomato sauce in oil increases the body's capacity to absorb an ingredient called lycopene. It lowers the chance of cancerous prostate growth and.

While lycopene does not contribute with cervical cancer prevention however, it can be linked to increasing the body's capacity to combat infectious illnesses which is why it can be helpful in the elimination of HPV infection. Sauces and juices made from tomatoes contain higher levels of Lycopene. It is suggested that tomato should be eaten in its fresh or cooked forms and not stored in cans since the packaging may cause pollution.

Supplements to diet

The majority of Americans within the United States have access to healthful foods, the usage of supplements for health is common across Americans. Research suggests that more than 50% of American adult consumers use nutritional supplements. Furthermore, 60 to 80 percent of patients suffering from cancer took dietary supplements prior to, during or following diagnosis and treatment.

Patients with cancer take supplements for various motives: aiming to prevent cancer; following the guidance of their family and friends as well as healthcare professionals; enhancing their immune system as well as being aware of the signs as well as side effects from cancer as well as its treatment.

It is the Dietary Supplements, Health, and Education Act of 1994 (DSHEA) describes supplements for dietary use as items that can be taken in a pill form and that contain "nutritional ingredients" used to add to the diet. The ingredients in food comprise minerals, vitamins and plants. They also include herbs and compounds such as amino acids and metabolites of enzymes and organic tissue. They are available in a variety of formats, including tablets, capsules and liquids, capsules, tinctures tea, extracts, powder, concentrate.

There's a lot of debate about supplementation during chemotherapy, particularly antioxidants. There is a possibility that supplements from dietary sources may interfere with cancer treatment, and possibly hinder the efficacy of the treatment is an issue. A few studies suggest that large amounts of vitamins and minerals that come from supplements could actually hinder the death of cancer cells as well as affect conventional treatments.

However, other studies suggest the opposite. Overall, the nutritional and protective ingredients found from whole food sources are better than those found in high-dose supplements.

The following suggestions from cancer experts are:

When using nutritional supplements:

Supplements for diet should not substitute for food items that are rich in nutrients. Consume a variety of plants-based food items, which includes at least five portions of fruits and vegetables that are not starchy each daily.

The use of supplements to the diet is not recommended in the prevention of cancer.

If you're planning to begin taking or have already taken supplements for your diet be sure to discuss all of the products you are taking together with your physician.

Supplements for diet may be suggested to you, and may be prescribed by your doctor to treat certain ailments including osteoporosis, for instance. anemia caused by iron deficiency.

Supplementation with nutrition should be supervised and supervised by the cancer treatment team.

Chapter 22: Sleep

With the knowledge regarding the vital importance of sleep for general health has increased numerous sleep researchers are now focusing on the ways in which sleep and cancer are connected.

Though more research is necessary but experts have discovered an interconnected relation. Sleep problems can be an indicator of the likelihood of the development of certain kinds of cancer. They also can affect the development of cancer and the efficacy of treatment.

Furthermore, cancer could disrupt sleeping. Cancer symptoms or adverse effects from treatment may interfere with sleep and impact the your quality of life who suffer from cancer. It can also trigger permanent mental and physical changes that disrupt sleep for cancer patients who have completed the treatment long ago.

Knowing the intricate links between sleep and cancer opens up possibilities to improve your the health of. Even though it's not possible to prevent the risk of developing cancer, a healthy sleeping habits can help reduce the risk element. In the case of cancer patients sleeping better can make people feel healthier mentally and physically as well as improve their capacity to deal with cancer.

Can sleep affect cancer?

Sleep plays an important role in our wellbeing. Due to its effect on virtually all body systems it is evident that sleeping can impact cancer in various ways.

Systems that may be affected by sleeping in ways that impact risk for cancer are the immune system, the brain hormone production and metabolism regulation and the body's weight. Sleep affects the functions of cells through altering their surroundings or the signal which affect the growth of cells.

Though it is still an emerging subject of research These sections offer an overview of the current research regarding the possible impact of sleeping on the risk of cancer as well as treatment.

Any person who is concerned about their sleeping or risk of developing cancer should consult their physician to determine what this means for their specific circumstance.

The effects of sleep on cancer and the risk of getting it

There is evidence to suggest that several aspects of sleep - the duration of sleep, quality of sleep the circadian rhythm, and sleep disruptions can impact the risk of developing cancer. But, research concerning this issue aren't all the time conclusive and reliable and could indicate issues with the accuracy of long-term data on sleep.

Sleep duration

The effects of the duration of sleep on the risk of developing cancer have frequently been inconsistent. Variations in the results could be related to how data on sleep is taken into account, the kind of cancers are included in the analysis in addition to how other aspects which may influence cancer risk are taken the equation.

The research has proven that people who rest less than six hours each every night have a greater likelihood of dying. the results of a large study showed that those who sleep less sleep are at a higher risk of developing cancer.

Certain cancers have been found to be prone to a shorter periods of sleep have been linked to a higher chance of colon polyps developing, that can turn cancerous. For older people, some studies have linked a decreased sleeping hours to a greater risk of developing stomach cancer. It also discovered possible connections between thyroid and bladder cancers, as well as head and neck cancers.

These studies, however, aren't conclusive. Sleeping less hasn't been associated with many types of cancer, such as lung cancer in the other research. A few studies have found lower cancer incidences in those who rest less than 7 or 8 hours per night.

In studies on animals, the lack of sleep has been associated with increased "wear and tear" on cells. This can cause DNA damage which can cause cancer. Though it's yet to be definitively observed in human studies however, it provides a possible method of connecting sleep with cancer.

Additionally, sleep deprivation may increase the likelihood for cancer. Insufficient sleep is connected to obesity, which is a proven danger factor for several kinds of cancers. Sleep deprivation is connected to issues with the immune system including chronic inflammation that can raise the chance of getting cancer.

Researchers also examined the long duration of sleep, which is generally considered to be at least nine hours each at night. The researchers found connection to the possibility of developing cancer. A study found that the amount of sleep required raised the chance of developing colon cancer among older individuals in particular those with a high weight or who were known to snore frequently. A long time of sleeping is associated with the increased risk of primary liver cancer as well as breast cancer. This is particularly true for the type of breast cancer in which estrogen promotes growth.

Sleep quality

The quality of sleep is typically harder to quantify accurately as sleep duration, in particular for long-term duration that can make it difficult to evaluate its effects on the risk of developing cancer.

In a research study with mice, disturbed sleep led to different forms of inflammation which promoted the growth of tumors and their progression. For humans, an observational study of over 10,000 older adults discovered an increase in the likelihood of getting cancer in those who assessed their quality of sleep as poor or fair.

A second study that surveyed over 4,000 women revealed a link between sleeplessness as well as triple-negative breast cancer. the most aggressive type of cancer. In a less-studied study, those who were suffering from insomnia were more likely to develop prostate cancer having the highest chance being those with the most intense sleepiness.

In the same way, as it relates to sleeping duration, additional research is needed to replicate and validate these findings. The future research will help to determine the ways in which certain aspects of the quality of sleep, like the amount or duration of sleep interruptions, influence the risk of developing specific forms of cancer.

Circadian rhythm

The circadian rhythm acts as the body's internal clock, which runs all day long. It's controlled by an individual section of the brain called suprachiasmatic nucleus (SCN) which transmits signals to all parts of the body in order to increase activity depending on the day's time.

The light source is one of the primary drivers for the cycle of the circadian, and that's why when people are there is no artificial lighting, humans rapidly adjust to a routine of staying awake during the day, and then sleeping once the light goes down. In modern times the constant exposure to artificial light as well as night shifts during work and the rapid travel between time zones may make a person's circadian cycle to shift according to the normal time of day.

An increasing body of evidence suggest that disturbances in the cycle of circadian rhythm could play an important influence on the growth of cancer. Circadian signals can be involved in cell division and growth which affects the way that DNA damage and mutations can take place. In addition, metabolism and hormone production along with the function of immunity are influenced by influences from the circadian cycle and could be affected by a wrong circadian rhythm.

The profound effect of the circadian rhythms in these systems of the body implies that disruptions in the circadian rhythm could have many possible connections with the growth of cancer which includes liver, breast colon, lung pancreas and ovarian cancer.

The practice of night work, also sometimes referred to as shift work is frequently a reason for the misalignment of circadian rhythms Shift employees are more at chance of developing cancer. It is believed that the International Agency for Research on Cancer (IARC) is a review of the available evidence and determined shift work "probably carcinogenic".

Certain researchers have proposed that there could be interplay between circadian rhythms as well as exposure to carcinogens30 which suggests that disruption of circadian rhythm can increase susceptibility to the risks.

Obstructive sleep anapnea

The study of the connection between cancer and sleep disorders has been largely focused on the OSA, which is also known as obstructive sleep apnea (OSA). OSA is characterized by repeated interruptions of breathing, which can cause fragmented sleep and decrease the quantity of oxygen present in blood. This is a condition referred to as hypoxia.

Studies on animals have revealed that sleep disturbances as well as hypoxia caused by sleep apnea can set the stage for increased tumor growth. Humans also, a variety of effects from sleep apnea could result in a cancer-promoting atmosphere.

These dreadful effects, which include the alteration of immune function as well as chronic, moderate and systemic inflammation the oxidative stress and sleep disorders, are caused by hypoxia. It could cause certain immune system to become less efficient in fighting cancerous cells. Low oxygen levels are present in a variety of tumor types and could indicate the hypoxia caused by sleep apnea can increase the risk of cancer.

In spite of these biochemical mechanisms that explain a link with OSA as well as cancer researchers are not able to provide general outcomes regarding OSA as an indicator of risk.

Indeed, multiple massive long-term studies on people who suffer from OSA across Spain, the United States and Spain have identified an increased likelihood of death from cancer among those with severe and moderate OSA. Studies of smaller size have revealed connections to OSA with breast cancer. The presence of severe OSA has been linked to an increase in the risk of prostate uterine, lung and kidney cancers and malignant melanoma, too.

But, not all scientists have found similar types of cancer-related risk or death in those with OSA Some studies have revealed fewer instances of cancer among people suffering from OSA. The differences in the research could be due to different methods of the measurement of OSA and the lack of data available on those who are receiving treatment for OSA as well as whether OSA is linked with other health conditions, like heart disease, obesity or diabetes that could influence the likelihood of developing cancer.

The effects of sleep on cancer and the progression

Sleep can play a part in the development and growth of cancer in the course of time. A few of the elements related to cancer risk like the impact of sleeping on hormones, metabolism and inflammation can influence the degree of aggressiveness in cancer but further research is needed to establish the connection.

Women with breast cancer, a study revealed that sleeping for at least nine hours each at night has been linked with an increased risk of death from breast cancer, as well as all other reasons. A second study revealed that sleep which was not in sync with the circadian rhythm related to faster recrudescence of breast cancer following the initial treatment.

A study that looked at colon cancer and sleep showed that those who experienced an infrequent sleep period prior to being diagnosed had a greater likelihood of death from cancer however, this study, as with numerous studies, only found correlation, and not cause.

Obstructive sleep apnea can also be considered to play a part in the development of cancer since sleep fragmentation and hypoxia can aid cancerous cells to grow and spread to different areas of the body.

Treatment for cancer, sleep and sleeping

Sleep patterns of cancer patients can impact their ability to respond to treatment for cancer as well as a deeper knowledge of the circadian rhythms could result in more effective treatment options for cancer.

Since the procedure of cell division and proliferation is controlled by the rhythm of the day and the circadian rhythm, cancerous cells could be more tolerant or resistant to treatment, based upon the time when treatments are administered. The majority of cancer drugs target enzymes, proteins, or receptors located on the surfaces of cells. The majority of them are affected by the circadian rhythm.

While still under development, the chronotherapy treatment is an element of treatment for cancer that seeks to maximize the effectiveness of chemotherapy, radiotherapy and immunotherapy in accordance with the rhythm of a person's circadian. Certain researchers believe that chronotherapy can help treatments eliminate more cancerous cells while lessening the harm to healthy tissues.

New drugs that utilize understanding of the circadian rhythm in order to combat cancer might also be developed. In particular, medications which alter cell growth "on/off" signals that are associated with the cycle of the circadian clock have been found as early-stage research has confirmed positive results in a variety of kinds of cancer.

Sleep quality can impact how patients heal and react to treatments. In particular, sleep deprivation has been associated with more discomfort, longer hospitalizations and an increased chance of developing complications for women who have the procedure for breast cancer.

The research on sleep apnea obstructive and cancer has shown that the condition may make certain treatments for cancer less efficient. Certain kinds of chemotherapy as well as radiation therapy perform best when the levels of oxygen in the cancerous tissue are high therefore breathing issues can hinder these therapies from performing at their best.

A lot of sleep-related questions are asked about it and risk for cancer

1. Do lights in the bedroom increase the chance of developing cancer?

Though not conclusive, some studies suggest that exposure artificial lighting at night might increase the risk of cancer.

The darkest part of the night is a key element for the circadian rhythm. It causes the body to release Melatonin, which is a hormone which helps to the sleep cycle. Apart from the benefits of sleep Animal studies have demonstrated that melatonin can fight tumors and repair DNA damage within cells. Therefore, theoretically sleep with the light on may disrupt regular circadian signaling and lead to conditions favorable to the development of cancer.

A study that examined the observational habits of subjects and their exposure to light sources and light sources, sleeping in a dark area was related to an higher risk of developing prostate cancer, but with a lower chance of developing breast cancer. In light of these contradicting findings that are not a good fit, more study needs to be done on the lighting that sleepers are exposed to in order to discover whether it's a significant risk factor in cancer.

2. Do you have the potential to contract cancer if you lie close to your phone?

There's no evidence to suggest that sleeping near the phone is a risk for cancer. The energy source generated by cell phones, which is known as non-ionizing radiation does not cause DNA damage; rather, the only evidence of a biological impact is that it causes warming. The studies of users of cell phones did not reveal a consistent pattern of an increased risk for brain tumors, or any other types of cancers.

While there's no definitive connection between cellphones and cancer, some doctors suggest that you not keep the phone close to your head for prolonged durations of time. In this regard, it is recommended to place your mobile placed on your nightstand or an open drawer.

Though it's not clear if this causes cancer, technological devices in the bedroom may disrupt sleeping, which is why if do not use your smartphone before going to your bed, it may assist you to sleep.

3. Do bras that are worn for sleeping result in breast cancer?

Wearing a bra while sleeping does not pose a risk for the development of cancer. One study did not find any connection between wearing bras with breast cancer risk and there's any plausible explanation from a biological perspective as to why wearing a bra could result in the mutations of DNA that are found on cells required to cause cancer.

What is the impact of cancer on sleep quality?

Cancer can trigger major insomnia, and can impact the capacity to sleep and remain asleep through the evening.

The estimates suggest that around half of cancer patients experience difficulties getting to sleep. Certain studies have revealed that there is a greater number of insomnia that resulted in nearly 70% of women suffering from Gynecologic and breast cancers experiencing signs of sleepiness. The incidence of insomnia is even greater when patients have advanced cancer. The rate is as high as 72 percentage

In addition, evidence suggests that the numbers could be overestimated because many cancer patients don't speak about their sleep issues with their physicians.

There are a variety of possible factors that cause trouble sleeping for patients with cancer.

1 Inflammation or pain caused from a treatment or tumor

2 Gastrointestinal and urinary tract disorders due to cancer or its treatment

3 Sleep disturbances during hospital stays

4 Stress, anxiety and depression which can cause cancer

5 Fever and infections may occur because from a decreased immunity during chemotherapy cough, or difficulties breathing.

Six side effects associated with medicines, like the effects of pain relievers, which can induce drowsiness, but also affect the quality of sleep.

7 Sleep patterns disrupted caused by daytime sleepiness as well as napping

Numerous of these issues can be a contributing factor to sleep disorders that can differ between individuals based on the kind of cancer, the treatment that was taken, as well as general well-being, which includes any co-morbidities.

The treatment for cancer may result in symptoms that are similar to various sleep conditions. When a study was conducted of more than 1,000 patients with cancer, a large portion said they were experiencing leg muscles that were restless, i.e. they were unable be able to stretch their legs when lying in bed. Certain kinds of jaw surgery to treat neck and head cancer could lead to obstruction sleep apnea that could necessitate surgery to correct the problem.

Sleep better and reduce the risk of developing cancer.

It is crucial for those diagnosed with cancer and having trouble getting enough sleep to talk with an expert doctor to discuss their signs, the cause and options. Because of the impact of sleeping on wellbeing, mood and mental health, a more restful sleep will significantly increase living quality cancer patients.

The use of medication and counseling can help promote the quality of sleep. Research studies in patients with breast cancer have proven the treatment of cognitive behavioral treatment to treat insomnia (CBT-I) is a method of trying to alter negative thinking regarding sleep, can improve the quality of sleep and mood, while also increasing immune performance. Combining CBT-I with medication may be more effective in enhancing sleeping quality and enhancing the quality of life.

This can also assist cancer patients to improve their sleep health, including their bed layout as well as their daily sleep routines. Some examples of this are ensuring a consistent sleeping routine, making sure that your bedroom and bed feel comfortable and relaxing while limiting the use of devices at night.

The importance of sleep and cancer prevention

The diagnosis of cancer can cause a range of life-altering changes. The emotional and physical effects of treatment for cancer are long-lasting and pose numerous challenges for those who have survived cancer.

The study looked at women who had breast cancer, from six months to five years following diagnosis, 78% of them had more than average sleep disturbances. They also noted that sleeping was among the top concerns that affected their overall health.

Sleep problems are particularly important for those who have survived cancer that was diagnosed in childhood. Childhood cancer and the treatment for it can have lasting effects which can affect mental as well as physical growth. A good night's sleep can mitigate those effects as well as boost your immunity system to improve overall health.

Cancer patients should consult their physician regarding establishing an overall wellness program62 that does not only cover sleeping, but includes various other vital health concerns like nutrition, exercise, as well as the aftercare . The plan could include measures for good sleep hygiene in order to promote healthy sleep routines.

Chapter 23: Avoid Sunburns

Skin aging is accelerated by sunburns. They can be a significant cause of cancers like basal cell carcinoma and squamous tumors,, which are among the deadliest kinds that cause skin cancer. It is completely preventable to get sunburns and avoiding sunburns can lead to wrinkled and the skin looking wrinkled.

UV rays, also known as sunburns that are the sun's radiation that can cause skin cancer, wrinkles, sunburn and even sunburn. Ultraviolet rays, commonly known as UV rays, can be divided into UVA radiations as well as UVB radiations. UVB Rays are responsible for the occurrence of sunburn. which cause sunburn. UVB is stronger and has a greater proximity in proximity to sun. UVA Rays cause early wrinkles of the skin. UVB is equally efficient regardless of the distance.

The sunburn is prevented through avoiding UVB sunlight rays by using any sunscreen with SPF 15 and up. It is recommended to avoid sunburn by keeping away from the scorching sunlight rays between 10am and 4pm. Also, be sure to stay clear of the sun's rays near the equator at high altitudes.

In order to prevent skin cancer and premature wrinkles of the skin, it is recommended to use sunscreen that has UVA as well as UVB defense, or broad spectrum of protection from UV rays that the sun emits.

The sun's UV rays can cause damage even in. Make sure you are protected with sunscreen to prevent skin cancer as well as wrinkles that don't appear until later even if the sun strikes the skin with a window.

Sunburn due to UVA can still be a possibility using a commercial tanning bed that reduces sunburn. You should wear the bronzing accelerator to speed up mylanin production on the skin. Apply a moderate UVA blocker such as SPF4 or 8. If you suffer from sunburn.

To treat sunburn, choose the product that contains Vitamin E as well as Aloe Vera This will help to restore the skin's elasticity.

Treatment lotion for sunburns can heal the injury by moisturizing your skin.

When you are walking in the sun, you can avoid getting burns by wearing an umbrella to shield yourself. The cause of freckles is exposure to UV rays from the sun as well as the damage to your skin. Do not dismiss freckles as normal even if they are as a group or an area that is new to the skin. Check for indications of skin cancer, especially similar to a mole that is changing shape. See a doctor and get it examined. Some clothing doesn't protect you from UV radiations from the sun clothing, cotton and light fabrics aren't protected from UV ultraviolet rays.

Chapter 24: Drink Less Alcohol

Consuming alcohol regularly as well as alcohol increases the likelihood of getting cancer. Alcoholic drinks have been proven to raise the risk of throat (pharynx) and mouth (larynx) cancer as well as breast cancer, colon cancer, liver cancer (colon and the rectum) and esophageal carcinoma.

The drinking of alcohol isn't the only thing that can increase the likelihood of getting cancer. In fact, even tiny amounts of alcohol drinks can increase the risk of developing cancer, however the stronger the beverage is, the greater the chance.

Consuming small amounts of red wines regularly can be beneficial to the heart when you are older, but there's no evidence to suggest that alcohol is a preventative measure against any kind of cancer. Cancer risk is the same for every alcohol-based drinks, such as alcohol, beers, and wine. spirits.

What amount of alcohol should be consumed?

To decrease the risk of developing cancer, limit consumption of alcohol to a minimal amount or completely avoid it. If you must consume alcohol, drink no more than two glasses per day, and then stop your all alcohol consumption.

What can you do to reduce your alcohol consumption.

1 Record it in your diary. Write down the reasons why you wish to quit drinking and allow it to serve as a permanent reminding

2 Establish boundaries: Create the limits, and you should also set drink-free days. The goal is for not having more than one glass in the days you are planning to consume alcohol.

3. Take your time drinking: Do not gulp while drinking. Take tiny sips of your drink and don't drink with a full stomach.

4. Do not keep alcohol in the home. Avoid the lure to keep a bar open at home, or even storing alcohol in your the home. If alcohol is more accessible more likely are you of consuming the substance.

5. Physical activity: Stay active and engaged with relevant issues, as well as not allow time for idle time. Develop a new skill, participate in community involvement as well as use this time to develop yourself.

6. Be aware of factors that trigger your symptoms. Any triggers that increase cravings for alcohol must be avoid. Activities, people, locations or events which trigger cravings for alcohol should be handled in a way that prevents an repeat relapse.

7. Consider alternatives. You can drink a cup or sparkling water as an alternative to drinking alcohol.

8. Create a strategy and follow your plan. Have plans to control your temptations, for

example, avoiding bars or having an responsible with a partner.

9. Say No: Be able to be able to say"no!. Say no in the moment in situations that entice you before weighing up how much you could lose by not drinking the beverage.

10. Check your mood: track your mood and research yourself to identify when you're most susceptible. Learn manage your emotions, such as sadness, loneliness and sadness. You should also be aware of excitement, joy, and fear. They are the conditions which make people gullible.

11. Help: Request help from friends, family or health professionals, and so on.

12. Don't give up. It is possible to fail when you try to end the addiction to alcohol. Keep going, stay constant, and adhere to your program until you are successful.

Chapter 25: Lose Weight

A person who is overweight or obese is more fat-laden than other body organs like muscles and bone. Being overweight can cause the risk of cancer, and can cause an increase in the rate of recurrence in the aftermath of the treatment.

Talking to your physician is crucial, however it can be difficult for certain people since they are ashamed they are subjected to discrimination due to the fact that they are overweight.

In order to shed weight, and maintain the weight off, it is necessary to modify your lifestyle as well as exercise regularly and adhere to your diet. Even small changes could affect the health of your body.

While not everyone who weighs more than they should is at an increased risk for cancer. However, it is crucial to be aware of the risk for cancer in order to make healthy choices. It is also important to be aware of the warning indications and symptoms you should be looking for.

Being Obese can increase the risk of cancer.

The relationship between overweight and risk of developing cancer is being investigated by scientists. The main reasons that they have found which increase the risk of cancer include:

1 The estrogen-producing tissues in fat tissue are produced that can raise the likelihood of developing breast cancer.

2. The weight gain can increase the amount of insulin as well as insulin growth factor 1 (IGF-1). Increased levels of insulin and insulin growth factor 1 (IGF-1) may aid in the development of certain cancers.

3. Fat tissue affects the ways your body regulates the development of cancerous cells inside the body.

4. Overweight and obese people with an increased belly fat percentage have a higher

risk of suffering from chronic inflammation and low levels, that increases the chance to develop certain forms of cancer.

The research shows that variations in your body weight over the course of your life can affect the risk of developing cancer:

Being overweight in the early years of a baby

Obesity as an adult

Obesity and weight loss repeatedly

These factors reduce the chance of relapses from cancer.

Consume a balanced and healthy eating plan.

Be sure to maintain your weight in a healthy range.

Exercise regularly.

Obesity is linked to cancer and being obese

Cancer of the neck and head

Thyroid cancer

Uterine cancer

Breast cancer

Cancer of the gallbladder

Colorectal cancer

Esophageal cancer

Prostate cancer

Cancer of the pancreas

Definition of obesity, and being obese.

The body mass index or BMI is a key determinant in determining the risk of developing cancer. It is calculated based on the weight you weigh and height. The calculation of BMI varies since it is influenced by body composition and race. BMI can be used to research the connection between obesity and cancer however, it isn't utilized as a measure to determine the condition of your health.

A healthy BMI ranges within 18.5 between 18.5 and 24.9. Any BMI that is between 25 and 29.5 is regarded as obese, while a BMI over 30 is considered to be overweight. Research has proven that people who have a higher waist measurement are at risk for chance of developing cancer and heart disease. A good male waist measurement is less than 40 in (101.6 millimeters) for males and less than 35 inches (88.9 cm) for women.

What can you do to keep an ideal weight.

1. Get more fruit as well as vegetables, whole grain as well as lean proteins within your daily eating plan.

2. Nuts are healthy fats that you can consume such as such as fish, olive oil and salmon They will that will fill you up.

3. Stay clear of foods that are highly processed, such as white bread cookies, chips, and packaged foods, which contain dyes, synthetic ingredients and sweeteners. flavors enhancers, and so on.

4. Do not drink sugary beverages like fruit juices, carbonated beverages and high-calorie foods as well as alcohol-based drinks.

5. Take 30 to 60 minutes of intense or moderate exercising or sports all week. Involving yourself in just the smallest amount of exercising can reduce your risk of developing cancer. As little as 5 to 10 percent of your bodyweight could reduce your chance of getting cancer by a significant amount. Ask your physician about your daily goal of calories burned to be.

6. The weight loss procedure is a possibility if you are suffering from heart disease or diabetes. Also known as bariatric surgery. The procedure is deemed to be as a procedure for patients who have a BMI greater than 35 or 40 and with a serious health problem.

7. It is possible to require medication when diet and exercise are not working and weight gain is leading to serious illnesses.

8. Talk to your physician for the most effective tips on how to keep the weight you are at. Weight loss and gain can be referred to as Yo-Yo diet.

Men who weigh more than average tend to be more likely to develop colon cancer than female co-workers

Chapter 26: Make Sure You Are Proactive And Undergo Regularly Scheduled Testing For Screening

Cancer is the most common reason for death that is second after heart problems. The number of cancer deaths is more than one million annually. The majority of cancer-related death could've been avoided by screening more people for cancer as a preventative measure.

Screening is a way to detect and treatment of cervical, breast lung, colorectal, or cancer. The colorectal and cervical cancers, as well as breast cancers account for 20 percent of all cancer-related deaths across the US in 2001. A timely diagnosis could cut down on the the amount of money spent on cancer treatments each year. The screening process is the very first stage in the treatment of cervical, breast lung cancer, as well as colorectal.

Cancer risk and screening

According to statistics, screening decreased deaths from cancer by at least 60%.

Additionally, mammograms taken every 2 to 3 years for females who are over 40 decreased cancer-related deaths between 20 and 25 percentage over a 10 year period.

In addition, Pap tests, which detects cancerous conditions in order to be treated. This has decreased cancer deaths caused by cervical cancer by between 20% and 60 percentage.

The statistics show that regular screening for colorectal cancer starting at 50 years decreases the risk of dying, and colorectal cancer screening can detect cancerous polyps that are precancerous, they are eliminated, the development of cancer is stopped. A regular colorectal cancer screening can reduce the risk of dying by as much as 60%..

Screening tests for cancers.

Screenings are available for kinds of cancer listed in the following table:

Cervical cancer

Breast cancer

Colorectal cancer

Lung cancer

Cancers of the neck and head

Skin cancer

Prostate cancer

Test for screening for breast cancer

A breast cancer screening test: during the test, a doctor examines the breast and traces it for any changes in the shape and the size of breast. The medical professional looks for any variations in the nipples as well as skin on the breast.

Mammography is a type of radiographic imaging that is designed to look and evaluate the breasts to detect early signs of breast diseases and cancer. The image of the test is known as mammogram. Mammograms may reveal tumors as well as various other irregularities in the breast.

Self-examination of the breast The breast self-examination is a examination at home that is done by yourself as you seek out or feel any changes in the breast. You should consult with your doctor in the event that you observe or suspect that you've noticed any signs of changes and seek immediate attention.

Imaging with magnetic resonance (MRI). It isn't often utilized to screen for breast cancer however it could assist those at a greater likelihood of getting breast cancer, especially people with a large breast or the discovery of a lump in a breast examination.

Cervical testing for cancer.

Pap test is a Pap test, a pathologist can identify cancerous or precancerous cells that are located outside the Cervix. The Pap test can be combined along with HPV screening, which is known as a pap test.

Human HPV (HPV) tests: The medical professional scrapes off cells that are outside the cervix to test the cells for specific types of HPV Certain strains put the patient at a higher risk of developing cervical cancer than other strains. The HPV test is more accurate and is performed with the Pap test.

Screening test for colorectal cancer:

Sigmoidoscopy: During this test medical professionals use the flexible tube, which is lighted and has an internal camera known as a an sigmoidoscope. It is used to examine the lower portion in the colon. It will look for parasites and cancerous cells. The test is not able to check the upper portion of the colon.

Fecal Occult Blood Test (FOBT) It detects hidden blood within the stool, which could indicate polyps or colon cancer. There are two kinds of FOBT are immunochemical and Guaiac tests.

The colonoscopy procedure it is when a doctor inserts the flexible tube of light equipped with an internal camera, referred to as the colonoscope in the rectum, to search for the presence of polyps, precancerous and cancerous cells.

Tests for stool DNA: These tests examine the stool for DNA in order to detect cancer. The test identifies changes in DNA from cancerous polyps and tumors in order to assist the determination of whether the colonoscopy procedure is required.

Double-contrast barium stool: This is an X-ray that shows the rectum as well as the colon following a barium enema. this enema helps to reveal the shape of the rectum and colon in being visible on images. This is a treatment option for those who are not able to undergo a colonoscopy.

Neck, head and oral cancers screening test

General checkups are the screening test to detect these kinds of cancers. The doctor will examination of the mouth, throat and nose for signs of malformations and also looks to check for lumps or bumps on the neck.

Dental exams are required for throat and neck cancers. Dental hygienists and dentists look for indications of oral cancers on your cheeks, lips, throat as well as your tongue.

Lung cancer screening test.

Medical practitioners use a low-dose computed tomography or helical (CT also known as CT or) scan to check for lung cancer. CT scans take an x-ray image of the body in various angles. The computer merges these scans into a 3D picture that shows abnormalities and tumors.

Prostate Cancer Screening test

Prostate cancer is diagnosed using the following two tests:

Prostate-specific antibody (PSA) test: This is a test to determine the levels of PSA. PSA can be detected in greater than normal levels in a person's blood when they have prostate cancer. An elevated PSA amount also indicates other ailments like aging or medical procedure as well as benign prostatic hyperplasia (BPH) and infection around the prostate gland ejaculation biking,

Digital rectal examination (DRE) A medical professional puts a gloved, lubricated hand into the lower rectum, and then examines the rear of the prostate gland in search of an increase in size.

Screening for skin cancer:

Skin self-examination by a dermatologist or medical professional examines the skin for evidence of cancer. This is a test you can perform the test on your own, and for areas that aren't visible clearly, like the back of your scalp or the your neck's back It is possible to ask an individual to look at those places to look for indications of skin cancer.

Dermoscopy:

Dermatologists employ a device known as a dermatoscope for assessing the form, coloration patterns and the size of lesions. This can be used as an early warning method to detect Melanoma.

Cancer screening is a risk.

Although screening may aid in earlier detection of cancer in an early stage, which will enhance the survival rate of patients, there's the possibility of risk. The risks listed below:

Screening tests for over diagnosis can reveal benign growths which are not harmful in your lifetime. However, individuals may get dangerous, costly and extremely stressful treatment that is not required.

False reassurances: certain tests for screening could suggest that someone isn't suffering from cancer, but they actually have cancer. This is known as false negative because this person might not receive the needed treatment in time.

False positives: Tests could show someone has cancer but in reality they do not possess it. This is known as a false negative.

Chapter 27: Reduced Risk Of Cancer Returning

Studies into exercise and diet suggestions for those who have been diagnosed with cancer in order to minimize or eliminate the likelihood of recurrences from cancer or secondary cancers as well as other chronic diseases are at an early stage.

There is no guarantee. But, recent studies of the population suggest health benefits for patients who are healthy in weight, follow a nutritious diet, and regularly exercise.

AICR Guidelines for Cancer Prevention and Risk Reduction. The AICR report as well as its regular revisions have found that survivors of cancer must follow the same exercise and diet guidelines to lower the risk of cancer.

The weight of your body

The research conducted in the past couple of years has revealed that being healthy and weight-wise is essential for those who have been diagnosed with cancer and to be as slim as you can without becoming overweight.

Healthy weight is believed to provide a biochemical which is an "anti-cancer" environment that inhibits the growth of cancer. The research has shown that carrying excess body fat, particularly abdominal fat that is too large increases your chance of developing certain kinds of cancer.

Consume a plant-based diet

Evidence suggests that dietary habits that focus on plant-based food will improve health and decrease cancer risks for people who survive. One way to achieve this is to establish an habit of filling minimum 1/3 of your meal of fruits, vegetables and whole grains, as well as legumes and nuts. Likewise, 1/3 or less includes fish, chicken and meats. This includes lean, healthy food items such as fish, poultry in addition to foods that are low in fat, such as dairy products and protein sources that are plant-based.

Get physically active

In the everyday routine Make sure you get at minimum thirty minutes of moderate activity every day. As you become more fit, aim toward 60 minutes. Make sure to include more exercise including brisk walks, within your everyday routine. Limit the amount of time that you're sitting, e.g. B. sitting in front of your computer or TV. The sedentary lifestyle can be an underlying cause for the accumulation of weight, being overweight and obesity. These factors increase the chance of developing various forms of cancer.

Reduce consumption of red and processed meats

Cut down on the consumption of red meat cooked (e.g. lamb, beef, pork and venison) in the range of 18 inches. or less every week, and avoid processed meats such as bacon, cold cuts sausage, and ham help reduce the risk of getting colon cancer. Since cancer patients have a higher chance of developing additional chronic illnesses including heart diseases drinking less red and processed meat can help improve general health.

Make sure to stay away from meat at least three every week. Try meat-free dishes like stir-fries and soups made from beans, such as hearty beans or burritos made of black beans.

Beware of alcohol-related drinks.

Although there is some evidence that links moderate consumption of alcohol to reduced risk of developing heart disease, this impact is not applicable to certain forms of cancer. AICR suggests avoiding even tiny quantities of alcohol. The consumption of alcohol increases the risk for colon and rectum cancers along with oral, breast, esophageal as well as liver cancer. If patients with cancer decide to drink, limit their consumption to one drink per day females and two drinks for males.

A drink can be defined as:

1. Twelve ounces of booze

2. 1.5 pounds of distilled 80 proof spirits 5 Ounces of wine

3. Stay clear of sugary drinks as well as high-energy meals

Studies link sugary drinks, such as the regular sodas as well as high-energy food items such as fast foods as well as foods that contain sugar and fat, leading to obesity, weight gain and overweight. In addition, excess body fat can be an important factor in the development of various forms of cancer. Foods that are energy dense include:

4. High-fat, high-calorie snacks

5. "Fast Food"-or prepared baked goods as well as desserts and sweets

6. Food items that are ready to go or meals which do not require cutting tools (spoon fork, spoon, or cutting board), e.g. B. hot hamburgers, dogs, French fries, corn chips, potato chips.

Avoid using tobacco products

In any form, tobacco is one of the main causes of cancer. Consumption cigarettes should be completely avoided. If you smoke or chew tobacco, smoke the hookah or tobacco in any way contact your doctor for assistance in determining ways to stop.

Beware of eating salty dishes and other foods.

Processing is done using salt (sodium) Ingestion of too much salt may be hazardous to your health.